Instinctive Health
Inspired Living

Instinctive Health Inspired Living

Awakening Your Innate Brilliance:
The Art of Creating a Remarkably Resilient Life

Leslie J. Rose

Cover design by Chris Molé
Book design by Julie Csizmadia
Cover photo by Bryan Mikota

Printed in the United States of America

ISBN 978-0-9966766-0-1

Please visit my website for upcoming newsletters and free booklet.

www.LeslieJRose.com
www.InstinctiveHealthandLiving.com

CONTACT:
Instinctive Health and Living
2305 Ashland Street
Suite C-139
Ashland, OR 97520

AUTHOR'S NOTE

Nothing stated in this book should be considered as medical advice for dealing with a given problem or concern. You should consult your doctor for individual guidance for specific health problems. This book is based on the author's personal experiences and written for informational and educational purposes only. Much of the information about longevity cultures is readily available in the public domain. No claims can be made as to the specific benefits occurring from the use of this information.

Dedicated to all seekers.

May the Great Mystery be illuminated.

May our true nature awaken.

To my Beloved,
who fills me beyond
the Beyond

CONTENTS

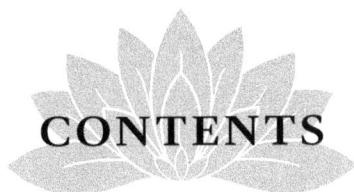

PART 4: APPLICATION AND REFINEMENT

PART 5: FOOD TRENDS, PRODUCT LABELING AND CONSUMER RIGHTS

PART 6: THERAPEUTIC SUPPLEMENTS

ACKNOWLEDGMENTS

I would like to express my deepest gratitude and appreciation to the extraordinary teachers, friends, family and companions of time, who – directly or indirectly – have helped guide my ever awakening spirit and contributed to the development of this book.

Heartfelt thanks to Chris Molé – Consummate book cover designer, whose perceptive insight and unflagging generosity helped guide this blessed project to fruition.

Many thanks to Carolyn Bond – editor extraordinaire, whose seasoned wisdom and encouragement gave me wings to fly.

Great appreciation for contributing copy editors, Patricia Florin, Courtney Williams and Carol O. – who each added their unique talent, flavor and craft to make the book shine.

Thank you to Julie Csizmadia of CsizMEDIA Design, for her beautiful creativity and talent in designing and formatting the book's interior layout and graphics.

A special shout out to Bryan Mikota, of Mikota Photography, for his wonderfully sensitive photography - on both front cover and interior photos.

And, to my exceptional son – *heart of my heart* – whose humanity and indefatigable spirit continues to carry forth the light of compassion and goodwill throughout the world – a deep bow.

INTRODUCTION

This is it. You've arrived. Welcome.

Take your shoes off, rest, and accompany me on a relaxing, entertaining and illuminating journey of self-discovery. For now, soften your focus on dieting, weight loss, exercising more, eating less and controlling or denying yourself. Simply allow the information to wash over you and respond to that which resonates with you.

Within these pages is a wonderful opportunity to explore and learn how to effectively tune in to your most unique and instinctive self – where you are in command of creating the most dynamically balanced and healthfully radiant body, mind and life you could ever imagine.

Accompany the author as she begins her 40+ year journey into the world of vegetarianism, natural-foods, alternative therapies, raw-foods diet, macrobiotics, meditation and the Eastern philosophy of energetic balance – culminating in a refined and applicable philosophy of self-awareness and attunement.

You'll explore the ancient Taoist principles of balance and harmony, the healthful practices of long living cultures, seasonal influences and adjustments, and ways to nurture and engage your own instinctual wisdom – that which is always present, always mirroring and always spot-on. You will cultivate a state of instinctually "knowing" the most suitable food, activity, climate or environment to shift, enhance and complement your current state of mind or body.

In essence, you will learn an effective, applicable and easy way to lighten up, ground out, get your mojo going, or just continue supporting your already balanced and harmonious state of being.

Let's begin with a little story...

Part One

My Story

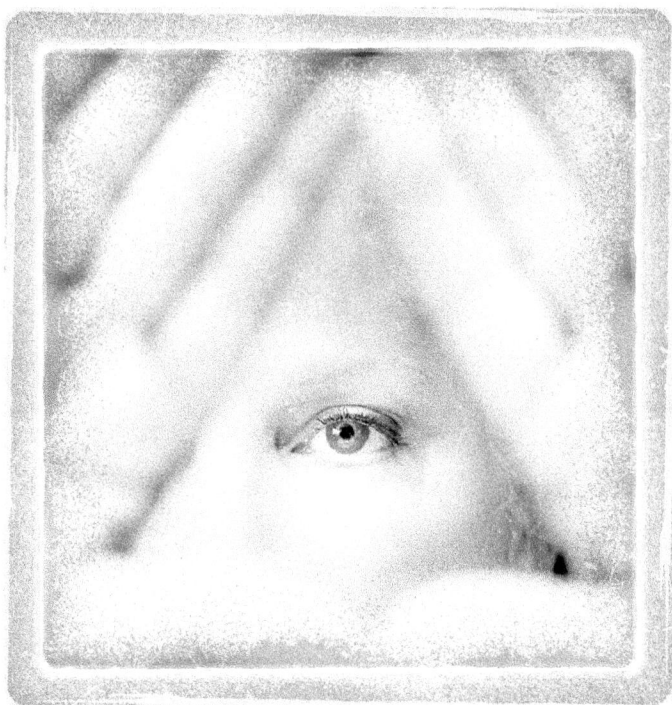

"Before enlightenment, chop wood, carry water. After enlightenment, chop wood, carry water."

~ ZEN BUDDHIST PROVERB

1

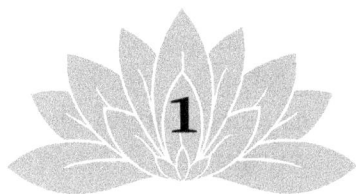

A New Philosophy

The year was 1971 and I was sitting in my senior high school psychology class. We were eagerly awaiting our guest lecturer – a previous graduate who was now living the "Way of the Sages." Word was he was going to talk with us about his personal journey into Eastern mysticism, reincarnation, karma and vegetarianism. Very cool subject matter, and I was more than intrigued.

From the moment he began speaking, I could feel a quickening inside, as if the atmosphere had somehow changed and everything in me was on high alert. As I listened to his stories and awakenings, I could feel subtle shifts in my brain, as if new circuitry was being connected that would allow me to see in a new way. I was transported to a wonderland that I hadn't even known existed – and I was eager to find out more.

After each lecture, I would replay the speaker's words in my head, mulling over his colorful stories and imagining myself in his place. As I vicariously journeyed with him, I kept experiencing a "reset" of sorts, as if my prior way of thinking would be forever changed. I remember going home from school and excitedly sharing this "new" philosophy with my folks, especially the part about vegetarianism. I told them I wanted to experiment with becoming a vegetarian and eating a more natural, healthful diet – just for a little while, to see if I felt any different or better. As foreign as this was to them, they had a live-and-let-live attitude, as long as it did not disrupt the family dynamic.

I carried out my experiment as unobtrusively as possible, continuing to eat my evening meals with my parents, while simply skipping the meat offerings. I still included the salad and veggie dishes, and also added brown rice with seeds and nuts as my main dish. As ordinary as this meal sounds, the simple combination of veggies, rice, seeds, nuts and salad would remain my staple for many years.

During this dietary transition, I became aware of a peculiar psychological phenomenon that occurs when a previously enjoyed food is suddenly taken away. There is a natural tendency to want a comparable replacement that will offer the same level of satiety and emotional satisfaction as the previous food. As a result, I started experimenting with vegetarian recipes that seemed to offer the main-entrée heft that I was missing. Now you have to understand that commercially prepared vegetarian entrées were virtually nonexistent at this time. The only prepared vegetarian foods available were from companies such as Loma Linda and Worthington Foods, which predominantly catered to the vegetarian diets of Seventh-Day Adventists. We are talking the early '70s, so the meager items offered were, in my opinion, tasteless and had strange textures and consistencies. By default I was forced to create my own homespun versions of veggie burgers, veggie stir-fries and veggie-nut casseroles, which, thankfully, got easier and better with time.

My family remained tolerant of my experimental eating regime and philosophy. Like many, they asked questions about the purpose of such a diet. For me initially, it was the idea of not needing animal meats in my diet. My rationale was based on the guest lecturer asking if we would actually kill an animal for its meat. For me, the answer was a swift and resounding "No." As odd as it sounds, I'd never really thought a lot about where meat actually came from. I mean, of course it comes from animals – but with names such as *hamburger, hot dog, bacon, ham* and *steak,* you were one step removed from the originating source. I had also never given much thought about how animals were raised or slaughtered. Their meat just sort of showed up in everyday life.

So, did I need to have meat in my diet – especially if I had to kill it myself? No, definitely not. That was reason enough for me to consider venturing down the vegetarian road.

This line of thinking prompted me also to question wearing and buying leather goods and animal byproducts. I applied the same line of thinking: Would I kill an animal just to wear its leather? Once again, the answer was "No." Well, talk about taking on a full-time job. I was discovering that animal products were in just about everything, and finding suitable alternatives was exceptionally time-consuming.

As a vegetarian, anything containing gelatin was out because it is derived from animal bones, hooves and skin. It is used in vitamin capsules, candies, ice cream, yogurts and even photographic film.

I began wearing natural fiber shoes, belts and purses. I even wore French "jelly shoes" made of plastic. (Talk about totally undermining any sense of fashion!) Anything that used gelatin in its making was out. Even today, gelatin is made from animal skin, tendons, ligaments and bones. Gelatin is also used in vitamin capsules, candies, ice cream, yogurts, and even photographic film. Avoiding animal derivatives meant no more boar-bristle hairbrushes or down jackets and sleeping bags. Even white cane sugar is filtered through charred cattle bones (bone char) during the refining process. Adjusting my life in this way became incredibly preoccupying and impractical. It didn't take me long to justify wearing and using the leather goods, hairbrush and down-filled products that I already owned. I decided I just wouldn't buy any new ones.

That commitment actually lasted awhile, until I got to the point I was spending an excessive amount of time being hyper-vigilant. I felt *owned* by having to check out every little thing that might have some animal derivative in it.

So after some deep soul searching, I became clear with my reasons for adopting such a lifestyle. For me, it had more to do with the healthful benefits of a vegetarian diet, as opposed to ethical reasons. The ethical aspect certainly played into it as far as eating meat was concerned, but I decided I would make a case-by-case decision about whether to purchase a product that had or might have some sort of animal derivative in its contents.

My engagement in this lifestyle continued to gain momentum. There is something very invigorating about doing things that can make you look and feel better. This was a practice that completely captivated me. It might have even bordered on obsession. I was continually on the hunt at vintage bookstores, searching for interesting, old-school books on vegetarianism, metaphysics and the classically coined "occult," which covered just about anything out of the ordinary. As you can imagine, 40-plus years ago, these weren't exactly prime topics of conversation, even among the most progressive of minds.

Mostly I found myself drawn to biographies where a turn of events – a "wake-up call" of sorts – had caused people to reexamine their lives. The wake-up call was usually preceded by a shocking health prognosis, which eventually led to a change in dietary habits, lifestyle and perspective. Understandably, most people were ill equipped when it came to making such changes on their own. Many had tried the conventional doctor-prescribed route of drugs, surgery, and sometimes chemotherapy, and often found the results sorely lacking.

Without a lot of preventative or restorative alternatives available, people were forced to blaze new trails – or suffer the consequences. They made radical changes to their former patterns of eating, thinking and living. They pushed themselves hard, experiencing both devastating blows and triumphant successes. These were the individuals who would become the early health-pioneers, with books, programs and practices that ultimately inspired a generation of "health-food nuts" like me.

During the time when I was still in high school, I frequented the neighborhood health food store and juice bar. A lot. There was so much to learn! I was like the blind person who now could suddenly see and wanted to behold every little thing.

Thankfully, the storeowners were kind and accommodating and shared much of their valuable wisdom with me. The more I understood, the more inspired I became. I had also begun hanging out at a Hare Krishna temple a few days a week after school. Although a seemingly odd choice at the time, this was the *only* place where I found like-minded people who seemed to embrace the tenets of karma, reincarnation and vegetarianism – the very subjects I wanted to know more about. I also found their Hindu philosophy, devotional chanting, philosophical discussions, meditations and shared vegetarian meals – well, rather engaging.

We would meditate together to "quiet our chattering minds." We would share wonderful tasting Indian vegetarian food called Prasad, the term given to any food that was blessed, chanted over or prayed over. As with many spiritual paths, it was considered highly beneficial for us to continually chant the sacred names of God. We were also encouraged to read and contemplate Vedic Holy Scripture (especially the Bhagavad Gita), to maintain a vegetarian diet, and to live as devotional a life as possible.

While the Krishna devotees served as a helpful support system at the time, it was destined to be relatively short-lived. My inner prompting and unquenchable thirst for greater knowledge kept spurring me on. During this time, I'm sure some of my friends were shaking their heads, wondering if I might actually join the group on a more permanent basis. That, of course, would entail shaving my head, donning a sari and offering the "good word" (and incense) to anyone inclined to listen.

Nope, I just couldn't see it. I don't think I had the necessary level of devotion for this particular spiritual path.

Shortly afterward, I began making some wonderful connections with like-minded folks at local yoga and meditation classes. It seemed that those drawn to these types of classes also resonated with eating and living more consciously. We would share our personal experiences with fasting, raw foods, juicing, sprouting, colonics – you name it. It was such a rich and fascinating time of discovery! This was not the kind of stuff we ever discussed in high school health class.

> "The greatest medicine of all is to teach people how not to need it."
> – SUSHRUTA, 600 BC

At about this same time, I began working at one of the local health food stores in order to further my natural foods education. I wanted to learn about the rich and multi-faceted world of supplements – every kind there was. This included vitamins, minerals, herbs, homeopathy, tinctures, flower essences and just about every health-enhancing substance you could imagine. This job was one of the early platforms that allowed me to successfully manage health food stores and food co-ops years later.

I continued to expand my knowledge and education by pursuing advanced studies in holistic health and integrative nutrition over the many years that followed. While this form of academia served me well, I would say that my most insightful and inspirational wisdom came from my own investigative experiences.

> "The only person you are destined to become is the person you decide to be."
> – RALPH WALDO EMERSON

The year following high school graduation, I went away to college in Tampa, Florida, where I continued to explore the realms of spiritual consciousness. I majored in Eastern religions, philosophy and the arts to expand and deepen my understanding. I wasn't exactly sure what I would do with such a major, but these courses kept me deeply interested and fed my spirit.

The esoteric booklist that I was exposed to during my studies included such classics as, *Siddhartha* by Herman Hesse, *Autobiography of a Yogi* by Paramahansa Yogananda, *The Way of Chuang Tzu* by Thomas Merton, *The Tao Te Ching of Lao Tzu, The Kybalion of Hermes Trismegistus* and *The Life and Teachings of the Masters of the Far East* by Baird T. Spalding. Each offered different nuances, insight and perspective on virtually the same subject – that of awakening the spirit. I was continually inspired and transformed by the stories of masters and gurus who had reached enlightened states of awareness that I could only dream of.

> "Enlightenment is absolute cooperation
> with the inevitable."
> – ANTHONY DE MELLO, JESUIT MYSTIC

I was also fortunate when, during my college years, an influx of spiritual teachers and masters from India came to the United States, and, as Providence would have it, many visited the University of South Florida campus. I had the good fortune to be initiated into Transcendental Meditation, to have personal audiences with the visiting gurus and to receive Shakti pat, a Sanskrit term signifying the sacred transmission of spiritual energy from the teacher to the student. I also traveled to some of their respective ashrams and spiritual centers throughout the U.S. and Canada.

Regardless of the specific master or path, the message was the same: Tap into your original Divinity and you would experience the connectedness and supreme Oneness of all life. This Oneness could be achieved or reawakened through the practice of meditation, self-inquiry, yoga, contemplation, sacred chants or prayers, right livelihood, a vegetarian diet and quieting one's "busy" mind and life.

"Sure," thought this baby spiritualist. "I can do this. I shall awaken my Higher Self." It seemed like a fairly doable proposition at the time, certainly given all the stories I'd read about masters – albeit mostly Eastern – who attained lofty, enlightened states while still quite young. I thought to myself that I, too, might possibly attain such heights. Indicative of my youthful naiveté at the time, I truly believed this could happen by the time I was 30. After all, that was 11 years away! Imagine my surprise when my 30th birthday came and went, and then my 40th, and still no obvious, sustained "enlightenment" to speak of – at least not the kind I had read about.

And yes, there was noticeable movement within myself, a progressive deepening and unfolding taking place on many levels. But I had been thinking that at some point there would be a kind of *boom,* and there I'd be – eyes wide open, mind suddenly clear, and the veil of ignorance lifted. Well, for me the *boom* never quite happened, or at least not the way I had imagined. Mine was a progressive path of exploration and practice – deeper exploration and more practice. Only when I looked back could I see how far I had actually come.

> "There are three stages in one's spiritual development,"
> said the Master. "The carnal, the spiritual and the divine."
> "What is the carnal stage?" asked the eager disciples.
> "That's the stage when trees are seen as trees and
> mountains as mountains." "And the spiritual?" "That's
> when one looks more deeply into things, then trees are
> no longer trees and mountains no longer mountains."
> "And the divine?" "Ah, that's Enlightenment," said the
> master with a chuckle, "when trees become trees again
> and mountains, mountains."
> – ANTHONY DE MELLO, ONE-MINUTE WISDOM

As time passed and my understanding broadened, my prior concept of enlightenment evolved. I began to see it as an ever-unfolding progression rather than an instantaneous occurrence. And, while this perspective still remains with me, I am and always will be open to experiencing an instantaneous and sustained awakened consciousness. Yep. I would love to inhabit such an unlimited state of being – all the time.

> "The only Zen you'll find on mountaintops
> is the Zen you bring up there with you."
> – ROBERT M. PIRSIG

Amid my esoteric college classes and the colorful array of alternative groups popping up everywhere, my college years were an incredibly rich and exciting time of internal evolution and external revolution.

"Wherever you go, go with all your heart."

~ CONFUCIUS

2

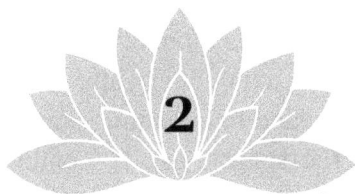

Raw, Vegan and Varied

When I first became a vegetarian, I elected to leave some fish in my diet for psychological insurance. As a newbie, I was not sure how the whole protein thing worked. Vegetarians and non-vegetarians alike shared a preoccupation concerning the subject of protein. It usually came down to the same question: "How do you expect to get enough protein without eating meat or fish?" Of course this was the early '70s and eliminating meat or fish from one's diet was not exactly commonplace. So, until I could figure the whole protein thing out, I decided to include a bit of fish in my diet. I began researching what it would take to completely eliminate all animal protein from my daily nutritional needs. As you can imagine, there were many differing opinions when it came to optimum protein consumption and utilization.

> "There is absolutely no nutrient, no protein, no vitamin, and no mineral that we know of that can't be obtained from plant-based foods."
> – MICHAEL KLAPER, MD

Two popular schools of thought stood out to me. One concluded that you could certainly do without animal protein but you needed to consume complementary grains and legumes at the same meal. In combining these food groups, each food's different and distinct amino acid composition (protein building blocks) would complement the other, thereby creating a complete protein – a superior type of protein that could not be replicated when eating the grain and legume separately. This diet of protein complementarity was explored in the 1971 classic, *Diet for a Small Planet* by Frances Moore Lappe. It was one of a few books at this time that actually explored and addressed a vegetarian's protein conundrum. She used supporting examples of indigenous cultures that instinctively incorporated these complementary combinations into their diets. Such cultural diets included corn tortillas and beans (Latin), rice and tofu/soy (Asian), chapatti and lentil dal (Indian), and pita bread and garbanzo hummus (Mid-Eastern).

Lappe would amend her position on protein complementarity in the 1981-revised edition of *Diet for a Small Planet,* believing that a well-balanced, nutrient-dense, natural plant-based diet would more than suffice for daily protein supplementation.

The second school of thought proposed that there was a pool of amino acids always present in the stomach, and when we eat a variety of colorful, nutrient-rich natural foods – leafy greens, root veggies, sprouts, grains, beans, nuts and seeds – we get enough combined amino acids from both food and gut to create any needed protein. No need to worry about specifically combining any complementary foods, just incorporate a well-rounded variety of natural foods. This theory particularly resonated with me, not only in its seemingly well-balanced simplicity, but also with reducing the ever-present emphasis on protein consumption.

As with most things, the more data I gathered, the more informed and discriminating I became. I continued reading about many longtime healthy vegetarians who apparently did just fine without eating meat. Six months into my vegetarian foray, I decided to eliminate the last vestiges of fish from my diet and see how I felt. I hardly noticed its absence.

It was quite apparent that being a healthy, dynamic vegetarian involved much more than just *not* eating meat. A diet filled with processed, chemically enhanced, sugar-laden foods had a very different effect on a body than one nourished by fresh and natural whole foods. Historical and scientific data showed time and again that a diet high in processed foods contributed to an overfed, undernourished and unhealthy populace.

> *It was quite apparent that being a healthy, dynamic vegetarian involved more than just not eating meat. A diet filled with processed, chemically enhanced, sugar-laden foods had a very different effect on a body, than one nourished by fresh and natural whole foods.*

I, like many, had been exposed to what could only be described as pasty, unhealthy-looking vegetarians who apparently eliminated meat but little else. I was beginning to realize that to look and feel energetic and healthy, it was essential to embrace a well-balanced, natural, whole-foods diet *and* lifestyle.

I was also discovering there was an amazing amount of diversity in the way people practiced (and mightily defended) their chosen way of eating. Every diet had an originating philosophy, corroborating evidence and ardent testimonials. There were all kinds of advocates: raw food, vegan, lacto (dairy), lacto/ovo (with eggs), non-dairy, high-protein/low carbohydrate, natural foods vegetarian vs. philosophical vegetarian (not health-oriented), natural food/organic meat-eaters, macrobiotic, Ayurvedic, food-combining, allergy-elimination and intermittent-fasting proponents.

Norman Walker's primarily raw and vegan way of eating was a dietary philosophy that especially appealed to me. His popular books, *Vegetarian Guide to Diet and Salad, Fresh Vegetable and Fruit Juices* and *Become Younger,* were about the proven benefits of eliminating processed grains and starches, refined sugar, dairy and animal protein, and opting for a raw, vegan diet. Well into his 80s and going strong when I was first introduced to him, he was a living testament to this philosophy.

I also resonated with Arnold Ehret's *Mucusless Diet Healing System.* As the title implies, this author believed that mucus-producing foods were the cause of most disease and discomfort. By following his specific dietary recommenda-tions, one could effectively heal most irregularities in the body.

Both authors championed a mostly raw, natural, vegetarian diet consisting of a diverse selection of fresh fruits and vegetables (and freshly squeezed juices) along with avocado, grain, seed and bean sprouts, kelp, herbs, nuts and seeds. Elimination and colon cleansing were also given great impor-tance, as well as intermittent fasting. The fasting gave the digestive tract a chance to rest, eliminate and rejuvenate.

Sprouts are the budding new growth of a bean, grain or seed that has been soaked and germinated, much like the seeds in our garden. During this process, the starchy bean or grain is naturally converted into an easily digestible, nourishing veggie plant protein.

I found it interesting that the commonly thought of "healthy" foods excluded from these diets were cooked grains, beans and all dairy products. I had read enough about the pros and cons of dairy products to understand its exclusion, but was surprised that grains and beans fell into this category as well. In Walker and Ehret's opinions, if you were to include whole grains or beans in your diet, then the most healthful recommendation is to first sprout them before eating. Sprouting is a relatively simple process of taking a raw starchy grain, bean or seed, and transforming it into a more easily digestible and absorbable vegetable protein. I experimented with sprouting garbanzo beans (chickpeas), sunflower seeds, pumpkin seeds and mung beans, and found them to be a tasty addition to my salads.

Both authors believed that grains, especially in their processed state, were not only difficult to digest, but constipating and resulted in the production of mucus. Those enjoyable and satisfying comfort foods, such as pastas, pizzas, breads, pastries, pancakes, cookies and cake, all fell into this category. This was supported by the seldom-considered fact that wallpaper paste and papier-mache paste are both made from the very same white flour and water used in these comfort foods. These foods have the same glue-like, binding effect in the intestines.

Fortunately for me, cutting down on these foods or eliminating them completely was a relatively easy task – probably because I was still young and with a decidedly undeveloped palate. I was also laser focused on incorporating into my diet "all things healthy" and culling the questionable. I was experiencing a remarkable improvement with the way I felt in my body, mind and emotions. My perception and experience of life felt heightened, clearer and synced-up.

> *All of those wonderfully satisfying comfort foods, such as pasta, pizza, bread, cookies and cake, are made from the same white flour and water used in gluey wallpaper paste and papier-mache paste.*

Natural food restaurants were virtually nonexistent in the early days of my vegetarianism, so eating out with friends at all of our previous haunts proved to be challenging. My friends continued eating the same way they had always eaten. The same way *I* had always eaten. They enjoyed burgers, hot dogs, fish sticks, sloppy Joes, barbecued ribs, fried chicken, French fries, soda, chips, dips, ice cream and so on. Compared to what they were ordering, my options seemed dull and bland, even to me. I also felt awkward, like I was now an outsider somehow, the defector. It was as if my new philosophy and chosen diet somehow broke rank with my friends.

> *Eating whenever and whatever you want is one of those liberties in life that you don't want people messing with – and consequently, carries a lot of emotional weight when challenged.*

Now that I was no longer participating in our previously shared food ritual, my friends started to question me and silently question themselves – leaving us both with an unfamiliar sense of separation. Truth was, when you feel healthy and dynamic, the way most of my friends did, there can often be little reason or desire to change your diet. I was discovering that eating whenever and whatever you want is one of those liberties in life that you don't want people messing with – and consequently, a subject that carries a lot of emotional weight.

I was getting a very good education on how to temper and adjust the rheostat when it came to sharing my newfound philosophy. When we're young, green and freshly initiated into a new exciting venture, it's easy to become overly enthusiastic about sharing "the way." We learn the rhetoric, defend our position and sometimes adopt a holier-than-thou attitude without even realizing it.

It would take me many more years of exploring, under-standing and evolving before I could embrace a more seasoned approach of simply walking my walk and chiming in only when invited.

"*From wonder into wonder existence opens.*"
~ Lao Tzu

3

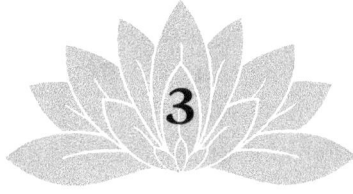

Out with the Old:
Fasting and Colonics

The importance of proper elimination and colon cleansing was a common theme in my readings, so I decided to investigate colonic irrigation. Colonics were similar to enemas, but the water was continuously infused (via the rectum) up the colon's entire length while simultaneously flushing out the refuse. This is in contrast to the enema's infusion into the lower region of the colon where the fluid is retained for a period of time. When the allotted time is up, the watery-waste is then expelled. The idea is to clean out any undigested or accumulated waste pocketed in the colon, thus allowing the body to return to its natural state of balance and efficiency.

I have to say, when I first got the you-have-got-to-try-this recommendation from a friend, my first thought was: "Uh no, don't think so." Doing something that involved *pooing* in front of someone, well, it felt just too awkward to me, regardless of its merit. In time, however, a few of my more seasoned friends chatted me up about the benefits far outweighing any perceived discomfort. I relented.

My first experience was a rather interesting one, on many levels. It took place in a clinical setting with a kindhearted and sensitive hygienist who quickly put me at ease. During the colonic and after, the unique sensation of literally having the *crap* removed from my body felt not only physically cleansing, but mentally cleansing as well. I was surprised at how different I felt.

> *Colonic irrigation is a process that removes accumulated waste, irritants, allergens and toxins from the colon. It is known to rebalance, rejuvenate and improve our whole-body well-being.*

Encouraged by my successful colonic experience, I was ready to explore the much-touted practice of fasting. Come to find out, there were several different kinds of fasting programs, each with anticipated outcomes or goals – both physical and psychological. Water-only fasts and fruit-and-vegetable-juice fasts are considered cleansing and detoxifying, resulting in a clearer mind and cleaner, better functioning body. A brown-rice-only fast is used for a more grounding and warming effect on the body. The psychological effect of this type of fast is believed to offer a more centered, focused state of awareness.

On a juice fast, the fruit or veggie, preferably organic, is juiced in its entirety – rind, stem, skin, seeds and all – as each part has its nutritional component. If a good overall cleanse is desired, the juice would be the only food or drink (water excepting) ingested for a three- to five-day period. If a deeper cleanse or detox is desired, a longer seven- to 10-day fast can be implemented. Consideration is always given to an individual's age, health, stamina and lifestyle when employing a fast of any kind.

The first time I was on an apple juice fast, I had not been counseled on quantity, and I chugged down a quart, *yes a quart*, of freshly pressed apple juice, not realizing that there could be some undesirable repercussions. Well, let me tell you what I discovered – a cautionary tale. When you've got a fair amount of enzyme-rich, high-sugar liquid interacting with pocketed or accumulated waste hanging out in the intestines – let's just say the combination produced a lot of volatility, cramping and discomfort. Having gas is always a drag, but this kind of intestinal distress was incredibly painful as well.

Unfortunately, I experienced this same objectionable occurrence a few times (*A few times?* you ask. Well, yes.), even when using *different* kinds of juice. I was under the erroneous impression that I could avoid another "gaseous" incident by excluding *apple* juice. That might have proven true, had I simply reduced my intake of juice – any juice. You see, I was continuing to guzzle fairly large amounts of juice to compensate for feeling physically and psychologically *deprived*. I was beginning to recognize a tendency that kicked in anytime I willingly (or unwillingly) gave something up, be it a food, activity or habit. My mind focused on what was missing. In this case, I not only had a food-deprived stomach, but an emotionally denied mind as well. Bad combination.

One of the biggest surprises for me with fasting was how much it magnified my emotional attachments and feelings of entitlement around food.

When I realized just how much my mind actually "ran the show," it was a revelation. This realization did not come to me overnight, but was revealed over time. I was able to see the mental and emotional patterning I had around eating whenever and whatever I wanted. And this was a pattern – a behavior that I found not only enjoyable, but also personally empowering. It was the idea that eating – and everything that went along with it – was *totally up to me.*

As with any routine behavior, I had not given it much thought until the pattern was altered. Fasting, dieting or prohibiting any habitual behavior causes the mind to experience a "pattern-interrupt" – a surprisingly unsettling experience. Take away any of our accustomed personal liberties, self-imposed or not, and there will be fallout, especially when it involves something we find enjoyable and satisfying.

In light of this revelation, I began to shift my focus from lack and what was missing to a more direct focus on the benefits of fasting. There were many. A practice or activity that could actually improve the way I felt, the way I looked and the way I performed, well, that was something I could easily get behind.

> *Our perception of the world is greatly influenced*
> *by our psychological lens and filters.*
> *By having a soft, curious and open attitude with any*
> *encounter or situation, we nurture a more refined*
> *and elevated consciousness.*

Along with my new perspective came the improved practice (thank God) of slowly sipping smaller amounts of juice. By slowly drinking smaller amounts of fresh juice, the volatile "fermenting" gut activity, and accompanying gas and cramping, were all thankfully thwarted. I began to eat my meals more slowly and consciously – with the intention of actually savoring my food. This simple redirect would contribute toward honing a much more refined and discriminating palate over the many years that followed.

A completely different kind of fast came my way while I was visiting a friend who lived in southern Oregon, which has a temperate climate, very different than my warm tropical clime in Florida. It was early autumn when I arrived and the daytime temperatures felt warm and silky. The nighttime temps, however, were remarkably cold, at least for this tropical girl. During one of our fireside chats, the subject of fasting came up, and we both shared our past experiences and revelations. She asked if I was up for doing a simple "acclimation fast" to adjust to the cooler evening temperatures. The instructions were simple. The fast would consist of eating in-season, locally grown apples and carrots for three days. I was to consciously and moderately eat only these two foods, in whatever order I chose and whatever amounts. I had never done an acclimating fast before. I thought I would give it a try and see what happened.

Compared to my prior juice fasts, this one was relatively easy – and surprisingly enjoyable. Because chewing was involved, I felt considerably more satisfied and didn't have the usual mind chatter that can accompany a fast. My mind was thoroughly entertained munching on the apples and carrots. It actually felt like snacking. What I found most surprising and impressive about this fast was it did precisely what was intended: I felt more "at home" and grounded in my new surroundings. My body seemed to handle the cooler evening temperatures as well – as if my internal "thermostat" was now working properly.

As my dietary philosophy evolved, my spiritual path kept pace. I found great affinity with those who were likewise drawn to the deepening practices of yoga, meditation, chanting, massage therapy, sweat lodges, alchemy, quiet contemplation and spending lots of time in nature. Being surrounded by those of similar ilk, who were also questioning the deeper meaning of life, inspired me to live more purposefully and consciously. The wonderful thing was the more I engaged, the easier it became to embrace the new over the old. It is said that it takes approximately three months of patterning a new behavior to effectively eradicate the old. And I was more than committed to making this my preferred way of life.

> "My destination is no longer a place, rather,
> a new way of seeing."
> – MARCEL PROUST

"When the shoe fits,
the foot is forgotten."
~ ZEN PROVERB

4

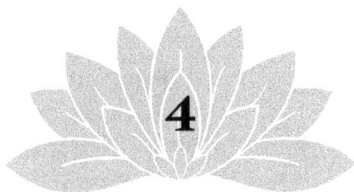

Environmental Influences: From the Tropics to the Mountains

In the mid-1970s I moved to Mt. Shasta after attending college in Tampa, Florida. During my four years of college, I had worked at a natural food restaurant called "The Natural Kitchen" and had saved enough money to explore possible living and working opportunities after graduation. Mt. Shasta ranked high on my list, as I hoped to spend more time with my spiritual mentor.

Mt. Shasta was a small town in northern California, where a four-season climate prevailed. When I arrived, I was very much the vegan, raw-foods enthusiast, believing these to be the healthiest ways of eating.

Throughout the summer months, I ate my raw food diet and conducted my activities much as I did while living in Florida. Even though I was now living 3,500 feet above sea level, my diet and lifestyle felt pretty much the same. Summer and fall were both filled with warm, sunny days and lots of outdoor activities. I drank my usual smoothies and fresh juices, and ate mixed-greens, veggie, avocado salads and fruit salads, and consumed plenty of dried fruits, nuts, seeds and sprouts.

As fall moved into winter, the changing rhythms of nature were palpable. Everything was drawing in and slowing down. The trees were losing leaves, activity quieted and evening temperatures dropped. And then, just like that, we were in winter. *Really cold winter.* As a young, energetic woman, initially I found it invigorating. But soon enough, the charm wore thin as I started noticing some uncharacteristic shifts within my body *and* behavior.

My first clue that something was noticeably "off" was an internal chill that caused me to feel peculiarly out of sorts and tightened-down inside my body. I had plenty of warm clothes and the house was centrally heated, but this sensation was originating from somewhere deep inside me. I also felt oddly unsettled, both emotionally and psychologically, which for me, was not only foreign, but also perplexing. I had no clue as to why this was happening, nor was I sure what to do about it. I had also noticed that my facial appearance seemed somehow different. Hard to explain, but it had a slightly fuller quality to it, like my usually defined cheekbones no longer had definition. Maybe I was holding water; I don't know. Not a typical occurrence for me. But neither was this whole thing.

As the cold weather continued, my standard fare of salads, fruits and smoothies quickly became *cuisine non grata*. In fact, the whole idea of eating refrigerated salads and cold smoothies was almost repellant. This makes sense to me now, but at the time, I was still aligned to the philosophy of a raw foods diet. However, what I was feeling had very little to do with "theory" and a lot to do with physiological instinct. I had a visceral, primal need to create internal body heat. The solution was simple. I would put aside my raw food ideology for now and heat the majority of veggies that I had eaten raw. I began steaming, sautéing and blending my veggies to make savory casseroles, soups, stir-fries, nut-sauces and hearty veggie stews. It was surprising to me how much better I felt eating this way – like night and day better.

> *Eating seasonal foods and aligning with nature's seasonal cycles promotes a well-balanced body, an even-keeled mind and a harmonious spirit.*

There was no comparing the altering effects of these warm, savory meals with those of my raw food fare during these cold winter months. I was amazed at the difference it made in my body and psyche. My belly was now satisfied, my body was favorably warm and relaxed, and I simply felt more at ease within myself. I felt back on track. Especially noteworthy was just how affected and out-of-whack I'd become from the persistent chill and lack of internal body heat.

As I look back, I realize that the feeling of warmth, in and around me, has always conveyed a feeling of emotional comfort and reassurance. Sunny days, soothing hot baths, autumnal warm colors, heated therapies, cushy socks, sweaters and scarves – all make me feel safer, easier and more secure within myself. Still holds true today.

This experience also made me aware of the equally important practice of physical activity during the colder months, something to get my body, muscles and respiration stimulated and my temperature elevated – something that actually caused me to break a sweat. One of the benefits of heating up the body and sweating is that it helps rid the body of excess fluid, which I was definitely holding. In retrospect, I can see how the fluid imbalance in my body contributed to a host of erratic, watery emotions. As to my altered facial appearance, well, after getting some fire back into my system (exercise and heated food), my "hidden" cheekbones had reemerged in all their well-defined glory!

> "Symptoms are not enemies to be destroyed, but sacred messengers who encourage us to take better care of ourselves."
> – FOOD MATTERS FILM

Mt. Shasta remained a richly rewarding and reflective place for me, especially during my spiritually formative years. Most of that had to do with extended periods of time with my cherished spiritual mentor, Sister Thedra, whom I had met in 1972 while still in college. Throughout the span of our relationship, I had the good fortune of living with her, caring for her and being under her brilliant tutelage. She was an intensely devoted, clear, generous and humble "Being of Light" (May 6, 1900 – June 13, 1992) who would have a tremendous influence on my heart, soul and life for many years to come.

5

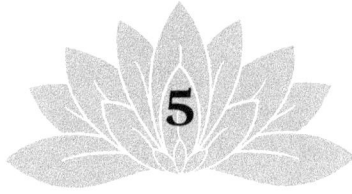

Macrobiotics in Boulder

I left Mt. Shasta at Sister Thedra's request. She had taken me aside one day and said we needed to talk. She kindly shared that it was time to leave the nest, explaining I had my "own light to carry" and needed to go out into the world and "be that light" instead of continuing to stay and take care of her. I believe her actual words were, "instead of taking care of an old woman like me." I was all of 21 years old and was rocked by her words.

To my young mind and spirit, I was "in the monastery" under the tutelage of the wise elder. I had not even *thought* of leaving. Had she not insisted, I would have continued "staying and serving" her indefinitely. With a tender but grateful heart, I left Mt. Shasta and Sister Thedra's side shortly thereafter. She sent me on my way with a few treasured books, some money, food and an open invitation to return.

I ended up in Boulder, CO, where I stayed with my brother while searching for some sort of health-oriented work. I landed a job helping to manage a small, natural café and juice bar, which operated within a natural food and produce market. During the warmer months, I continued to eat a raw food diet of super-food smoothies, mixed fruit salads with nuts, fresh pressed juices and veggie salads with sprouts, nuts, seeds, dulse powder, nutritional yeast, tamari, lemon and avocado. During the cooler evenings, I included a variety of steamed veggies and a bowl of brown rice or millet with the usual splash of tamari (naturally fermented soy sauce).

I discovered that the trick to making food "entertaining" as well as enjoyable is in adding well-seasoned sauces and dressings. This can turn a ho-hum meal into one that is enticing and zesty. The same is true for salads. All I needed to do was find (or make) some sort of tasty salad dressing that could also go atop cooked veggies. Finding the right seasonings and sauces is a critical step in avoiding the veggie doldrums.

At that time in Boulder, quinoa had yet to make its appearance on the local food scene. It would be another 34 years before this noble grain would reach the mainstream popularity of today.

While working at the café, opportunities came my way to volunteer for various spiritual retreats held in the mountains above Boulder, such as assisting with meal preparation in exchange for tuition. It was at one such retreat with a group called "The New Troubadours" from the Findhorn spiritual community in northern Scotland – that I met my future husband. He was a vegetarian and we shared similar philosophies regarding spirituality, life and love. He lived in Denver and I was in Boulder, and our relationship continued to deepen and develop over the many months that followed. We married the following year and chose the auspicious date of 7/7/77 for our wedding, held at our ranch in Golden, Colorado. Our beloved son entered the world in 1978, healthy, happy and cherished.

My diet remained primarily the same during my pregnancy, with some additional prenatal supplements and increased superfoods such as spirulina and chlorella. I did, however, have the occasional cravings for some nurturing "mama food," such as eggplant Parmesan, wholegrain pasta and cheesy casseroles. I gladly accommodated these cravings and found little if any downside, physically or psychologically. And, while these meals were very satisfying, they would remain a rarity because of their unaccustomed richness.

I was a young and healthy 23-year-old and found being pregnant a wondrous and enjoyable experience.

It was during this same year that my initial introduction to macrobiotics was made. With just a superficial understanding of it, and virtually none of the overarching philosophy, my first impression was that a macrobiotic diet seemed rather lifeless as compared to the predominantly fresh veggies, sprouts, nuts, seeds and fruits that I was accustomed to. In actuality, the foods in both diets were surprisingly similar.

It was the emphasis on a primarily grain-based cooked diet that registered to me as different. Where I had been consuming fresh fruit and veggie juice, salads and smoothies, raw seeds and nuts, and sprouted most of my grains and beans, those of the macrobiotic persuasion cooked, baked, toasted and fermented those *very same foods*. They also added seaweed, miso and some occasional fish.

The interesting thing was, as committed as I was to my raw foods philosophy, the individual who introduced me to macrobiotics was just as committed to his. As with any set of beliefs, there are varying gradations of understanding and perspective. During our initial discussions, we each shared our personal experiences, thoughts and opinions. These were not the easiest of conversations and not dissimilar to religious or political factions defending their respective position. Many times we just had to agree to disagree.

In retrospect, I think it rather funny on my part, shortsighted really, that I needed to defend or somehow champion the raw food approach, especially on the heels of my Mt. Shasta experience. How do you argue the merit between an apple and orange when you've only ever experienced the apple? I knew *nothing* about the actual philosophy behind macrobiotics.

I wasn't looking to adopt yet another diet as much as gain an understanding of how different environments and foods affect us physically and emotionally.

As the months went by, I was aware of a very persistent niggle that would flit in and out. It had to do with macrobiotics, that the subject needed a deeper examination. As the niggling continued, I found myself curious about checking out some previously recommended books on macrobiotics. I was surprised to find that it was a much bigger movement than I had originally thought. There were numerous books on macrobiotic principles, macrobiotic disease prevention and macrobiotic cooking. Again, I wasn't looking to adopt yet another diet as much as broaden my understanding of what had actually occurred during those winter months in Mt. Shasta. Could macrobiotics hold some answers to these questions of mine?

It didn't take long to find what I was looking for. There was plenty of information regarding the energetic properties surrounding food, climate, bodily environment, temperature and activity, and how each affects us physically and psychologically. According to this philosophy, the climate where a food is grown, the way it is prepared and the energetic properties inherent within each food, all have an influence on our body and brain chemistry. I could feel a quickening as I read this and realized I was onto something, and that excited me.

> *According to this philosophy, the climate where a food is grown, the way it is prepared and the energetic properties within each food, all have an impact on our body and brain chemistry.*

As the days and weeks passed, I dug deeper into this philosophy with a passion that matched my initial quest into vegetarianism. I wanted to find out where, when and with whom this philosophy originated.

I was surprised to read that the earliest recorded use of the term "macrobiotics" can be found in the writing of Hippocrates, who in his day (460-370 B.C.) was considered something of a medical maverick. It was only later, long after his death, that he became known as the Father of Western Medicine. In his essay "Airs, Waters, and Places," he introduced the word macrobiotics, describing people who were healthy and long-lived. The term originated from the Greek language, with *macro* meaning great and *bios* signifying life. *Great Life.* I liked the sound of it and what it implied.

Hippocrates theory of physis[1] described the reciprocal relationship between a living organism and its environment. He determined that all disease was simply "life out of balance with one's environment." He had observed that our health and well-being were greatly influenced by our environment, the changing seasons and our lifestyle and daily routine.

Bingo. This was all making a lot of sense to me, and I found myself wanting to understand more.

> *The genesis of macrobiotics was not so much a diet as a philosophical approach to experiencing a balanced and healthy life.*

As I continued researching, up popped the Greek physician and philosopher, Galen (c129-210 A.D.), who lived about 600 years after Hippocrates. Influenced by Hippocrates' earlier principles, Galen developed his own unique philosophy, called *dietetics*. Dietetics was "the practice of living naturally, organically and in harmony with one's environment." There it was again. I was starting to see a theme here. Galen also discovered that a plant's nutritional attributes could be positively or negatively influenced, depending on the quality of soil where it grew. Now, this concept may seem fairly accepted today, but we're talking 1,800 years ago.

Moving along, in 1796, the German physician Christopher W. Hufeland (1762-1836) published his book on diet and health, *Macrobiotic, The Art of Prolonging Human Life*. Hufeland also embraced much of Hippocrates' earlier philosophy on natural healing, and much like Galen, continued developing his own expanded philosophy of the reciprocity and harmonizing relationship between man and his environment. He used the term "macrobiotic" to describe the "science" of prolonging and perfecting life. As did the others, he considered the prescribed way of living in harmony with one's environment to be through a mostly vegetarian diet, intellectual stimulation, regular exercise and a positive attitude. These practices not only prevented illness, but promoted health, harmony and longevity as well.

Now, as far as I could see, none of these great pioneers were focused solely on the dietary aspect of life. To their credit, each of them practiced a systematic approach to living a balanced and healthy life, an approach that suited and supported an individual's body, lifestyle and temperament, rather than a one-size-fits-all formula. Each practitioner had taken the wisdom of his predecessor and fashioned it into his own. This was precisely what I wanted to do.

Next on the scene was the Western-trained Japanese military doctor Sagen Ishizuka (1850-1910). His philosophy of nutrition and health was called "Shoku-Yo," translated as "Food Cure" and based on the classic texts of traditional Chinese medicine. It was here with Dr. Ishizuka's originating philosophy that I believe our modern macrobiotic movement was founded. In contrast to the much-preferred Western diet prevalent in Japan at the time, Ishizuka's recommendation of eating a more traditional diet of brown rice, seasonal vegetables and sea-vegetables – with little to no animal products – was not favorably embraced or received by the Japanese general public. This was of little concern to Ishizuka, as the populace he served were patients who had been deemed incurable by the medical establishment and sent home with little hope of recovery. They came en masse to be assessed by him and receive his recommendations and wisdom.

Dr. Ishizuka's philosophy was based on two simple principles: First, that human health and longevity are dependent on the proper ratio and balance of the mineral salts potassium and sodium in the body (expressed as Yin and Yang aspects);

and second, that food and diet, along with geography, climate and physical activity, are all determining factors in creating and maintaining a healthy functioning and disease-resistant body.[2] The achievement of effectively helping to cure hundreds of patients through his dietary healing program was unparalleled at the time and contributed greatly to his reputation and acclaim.

The Japanese philosopher Georges Ohsawa (1893-1966) credited Ishizuka's philosophy and dietary recommendations with curing his own youthfully inherited tuberculosis.[3] Similar to the pioneers that came before him, Ohsawa was able to expand upon Ishizuka's healing philosophy with his own tenets for living a truly healthful life. His book, *Zen Macrobiotics*, published in the late 1950s, was very well received. He believed by following the philosophy he outlined, a person could readily achieve a healthful, balanced and contented mind, body and life.

The healthful indicators of a balanced mind, body and life, according to Ohsawa, were as follows:

- Embodying vitality
- Possessing an appetite for food and life
- Sleeping deeply and peacefully
- Enjoying a sharp mind and clear memory
- Appreciating good humor
- Exemplifying an appreciative attitude
- Living in accordance with the laws of nature
- Discerning and implementing right action

Ohsawa believed that "food was the key to health" and "health was the key to peace." His book helped raise public awareness about the prospect of living a "true and authentic macrobiotic life." He spent the better part of his life teaching and spreading his philosophy throughout Japan, Europe and the U.S.

Shortly after World War II, in 1949, a student of Ohsawa's, Michio Kushi (1926-2014) emigrated to the U.S. from Japan. His future bride-to-be, Aveline, arrived in the U.S. from Japan in 1951. They studied separately with Ohsawa in Japan, met after coming to the U.S. and soon married. Using Ohsawa's philosophy as their primary platform, they engineered a thoughtful, applicable, contemporary approach to the macrobiotic philosophy that was geared toward the Western-oriented culture and mindset. Their contributions became the gold standard of macrobiotics in the field of alternative health, whole foods education, disease preven-tion, holistic healing practices and macrobiotic cooking for more than 60 years. Without question, Michio and Aveline Kushi stimulated the greatest insights and inspiration within the modern-day macrobiotic movement.

I was impressed with the rich and diverse history surrounding this philosophy. It was fascinating how the original concept of "living in harmony with one's environment" expanded and morphed over the centuries. I was continually inspired and elevated whenever I read about these powerfully inno-vative pioneers, whose experiences, struggles and triumphs took them to new heights of awareness.

One such book was *Recalled by Life* by Anthony Sattilaro, MD. It was an easy read about a traditionally trained doctor, who in his prime, during his 47th year, finds out his body is riddled with cancer. The year is 1978 and having practiced medicine for more than 20 years, he decides to follow the commonly prescribed treatment of his doctors and hopes for the best. After his prognosis and accompanying treatment, he finds himself driving along the highway and notices two young guys hitchhiking. For reasons unknown to him at the time, he is curiously compelled to pick them up.

After introductions are made, conversation unfolds easily, and once again he feels uncharacteristically prompted to tell them about his cancer and remedial treatment. It just so happens these guys are health food advocates and recent graduates of a natural foods cooking school. They believe diet and lifestyle can influence health and disease, and by making positive changes in both areas, significant improvement can be experienced. *"Out of the mouth of babes,"* thinks the well-educated doctor, and he bids them adieu and promptly forgets about their encounter.

Months later, when his pain and condition have worsened to an almost unbearable state, he recalls his encounter with the young men. With very few options available, he decides to check out a natural, whole foods diet, and dives into the unknown world of macrobiotics. The book follows his frustrating and illuminating journey, as he explores new ways of thinking, eating and living – all while on his ultimate path toward recovery.

Three years after his original diagnosis, in 1981, the doctor is considered free from cancer and in remission. As a result, he becomes one of the most prominent physician advocates for the effective use of diet against cancer.

Years later, out of curiosity, I did a follow up on Dr. Sattilaro's progress. His cancer had returned in 1989 – 11 years after his terminal prognosis of 18 months to live. Sorry to say, his is not an uncommon occurrence in the fight against cancer, irrespective of diet, method, practice or medicine.

"I lived the perfect formula for cancer – a high fat diet, plenty of refined flour products, an insatiable sweet tooth and a generally sedentary lifestyle."
    – DR. ANTHONY SATTILARO

Part Two
Dietary Reformation:
Traditional, Industrialized
and Organic

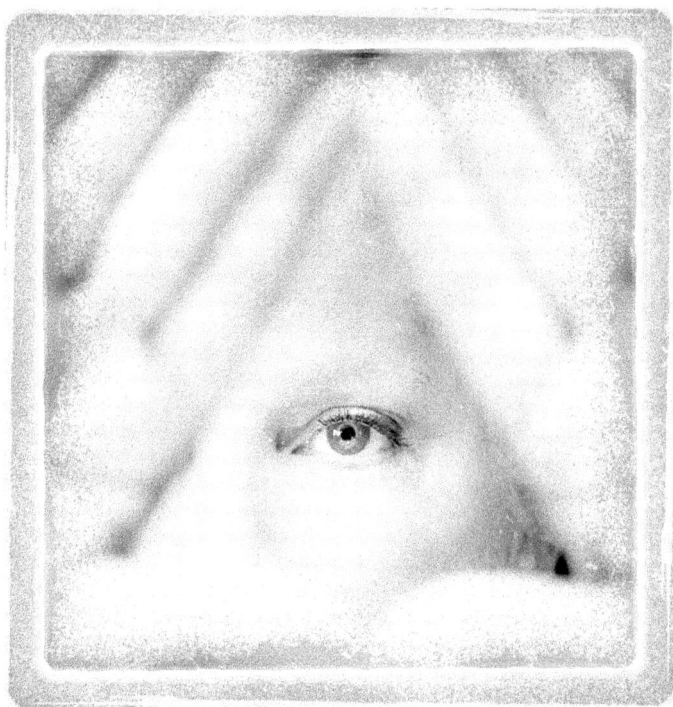

*"Understand the roots
and the branches
make sense."*

~ TAOIST PROVERB

6

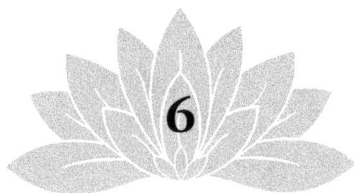

Food Becomes a Commodity

As I continued to educate myself about natural foods and eating healthfully, I was finding there was so much to learn. I was not following a diet as it is typically defined, where you are given specific foods to eat and others to stay away from. I had to figure out all the details of eating a natural, whole foods diet as I went along, which oftentimes felt like a crapshoot. There were parameters and gradations that I almost had to intuit, especially when it came to which products were truly healthy and which were considered marginal or verboten. This required personal education, continual experimentation and superior label-reading acumen – and even then I was subject to blunders.

I remember early on, when I was in high school, just weeks after I started the raw vegan diet, I heard about the wonders of carrot juice. It was mentioned lightly, thrown into a conversation about amazingly healthy foods to include in one's diet. So there I was, days later, at the grocery store, perusing the shelves, and what do I find? A can of carrot juice! I scooped it up and excitedly brought it home to have with my dinner. *Oh. My. God.* Worst tasting stuff I had ever had. Liquid, bitter, tinfoil taste, if you can imagine. How was I to know the only way to drink carrot juice and have it taste good, was freshly pressed? After that I became much more discerning with my spontaneous experiments. I decided to stick to the recommendations of more experienced people, at least until I had more time (and wisdom) under my own belt.

As my research continued, I was realizing that the more I found out, the more limited my options became. Even with so-called health foods, I had to assume that if items were prepackaged, boxed, bottled, dehydrated or frozen, then *some* sort of processing was involved. Once I had figured out a product's ingredients and level of processing, I had a decision to make – good, bad or indifferent? I could continue eating that food, eliminate it altogether or eat it only on occasion. I started wondering how we ended up going from the more traditional farm-to-table way of eating to this urban, industrialized process. Reasonable question.

In the early 1900s, our industrial food revolution began. It was a time of promise, when the prospect of bettering one's life was on everyone's mind. As a result, people began to move off the farm and into the cities, where industry was rapidly gaining momentum. Factories were in full throttle, replicating many of the farm-produced food staples previously found on farm stands and grocery store shelves.

As a result, newer and more progressive technologies were implemented for better, faster and more economical food production. Food manufacturers wanted to effectively address production costs, quality, appearance, taste, shelf life, availability and consumer convenience – all while increasing revenue. That was a very tall order, especially when it came to product stabilization and spoilage. Food manufacturers had to figure out ways to alter the natural progression of food's three-stage cycle of growth, "bloom" and decomposition. Scientists needed to discover how to sustain the "bloom" period and eliminate the decomposition phase. For that to happen, they would need to establish a method to remove the "natural life force" that gives food its appealing freshness, taste, texture, appearance and nutrition. Cue the so-called food scientists, whose task it was to find effective solutions. Over the next several years, they formulated and refined chemical additives, synthetic sweeteners, texture enhancers, artificial flavorings, preservatives and colorings – all engineered to fool and control Mother Nature. The concept was not a whole lot different in theory to the embalming process of preserving a cadaver, except that these newly formulated ingredients were deemed safe for human consumption.

But were they?

> *Food manufacturers had to figure out ways to alter the natural progression of food's three-stage cycle of growth, "bloom" and decomposition. Scientists needed to sustain the "bloom" period and eliminate the decomposition phase. For that to happen, they would remove the "natural life force" that gives food its appealing taste, texture, appearance and nutrition.*

One of the ways the "continual bloom" (or extended shelf-life) was sustained with wheat flour products was by removing the bran (outer protective hull) and the nutritious germ (the inner core). The remaining grain was then pulverized and bleached into sanitized white flour, which accomplished the desired goal of lasting months without going rancid. A food has to be pretty darn stripped-down to remain *that* well preserved. And, if it was that sanitized, was there any nutritional value left? Not to my thinking. But the food scientists had a quick fix for that.

After removing the nutritional constituents from the grain during processing (especially the valued B vitamins), a miserly few nutrients were added back into the barren flour, which was then labeled "enriched." Problem was, this newly stripped, non-nutritive, starchy flour now registered in the body as pure sugar!

For the general public, enriched flour became the norm. Most consumers thoroughly enjoyed these new wonderful flour products without giving it a second thought – so much so that the average person today consumes an approximate 138 pounds of flour products each year.[4] That is an awful lot of bread, pasta, cake and cookies. Given the statistics, we can assume that the average person will *continue* eating and enjoying these flour products, regardless of nutritional content.

So what do we do with all this information? Here is how I frame it: Understanding that the very same flour is used in both wallpaper paste and all those wonderfully rewarding, comfort foods, let's just consider ourselves educated as to what these flour products really are – entertainment food! In viewing them this way, we can be straight with ourselves and put these delightfully appealing cakes, breads, pizzas, crackers, pastas and cookies into the strictly "entertainment" category – and partake consciously *and in moderation.*

Another technology created at the time of our industrial food revolution was that of hydrogenating oils. Funny thing was, hydrogenated oil was first created in 1903 for soap. It was sometime after 1914 that the hydrogenation process gained great momentum with larger food companies because products could remain on shelves for months at a time without spoiling. The process involved extracting naturally occurring oil from soybean, corn, palm or coconut, putting it under severe heat and pressure, and adding chemical catalysts. This transformed the oil's molecular structure, changing it from a liquid to a thicker, semi-solid or solid form, such as Crisco or margarine. Given that this process addressed the inconvenient rancidity factor, hydrogenated oils were now used in making baked goods, snack foods, fried foods, non-dairy creamers and margarine-type spreads.

As farfetched as it sounds, this hydrogenated oil was much closer in its molecular structure to plastic than to oil – in fact, one molecule away. Consequently, our body is unable to process or use this foreign substance, which should be no surprise. The coagulated greasy fat causes a thickening of the blood's viscosity, causing it to coat and clog the arteries and blood vessels. It also causes additional strain on the heart as it pumps this thickened, sludgy blood throughout the body. Hydrogenated oils, also known as trans-fats, would become one of the greatest contributors in the escalation of heart attacks, high blood pressure, arterial sclerosis (hardening of arteries) and other cardiac-related complaints among the general populace.

Animal farms were also included in big agri-business' seeming "master plan." With the growing demand for meat, milk and eggs, growth hormones were now added to the feed of cows, livestock and chickens to increase size, weight and production, which once again, translated to increased revenue.

Antibiotic cocktails were also being used in great quantity to stave off the rampant diseases now found in the crowded, controlled, factory-farmed animal environment. As the consumer ingested the meat, dairy and eggs of these commercially raised animals, they also ingested the hormones and antibiotics that were injected into the animals. One of the challenges with these developing technologies was the lack of pertinent information to the consumer regarding the possible hazards of ingesting not only excessive amounts of hormones and antibiotics, but also other foreign chemicals, drugs and artificial ingredients into the body.

Moreover, as the momentum of these practices built, a consensus grew among larger agri-business and food-production companies that monetary profit, by all rights, took precedent over the health and welfare of the consumer. Without our knowing it, doors slammed shut and lips sealed concerning the candid disclosure of farming practices, food production, product ingredients and labeling. Such transparency was no longer required, nor proffered.

> *Organic foods are grown without toxic pesticides, herbicides and fungicides. They are grown without synthetic hormones or antibiotics. They are grown without genetically modified organisms (GMOs). They are free of artificial preservatives or chemical additives. Doesn't it make sense to eat organic foods whenever possible?*

Since then, numerous studies have connected the use of antibiotics and hormones in animal meats and by-products with human immune dysfunction, antibiotic resistance, allergic reactions and hormonal irregularities. There are cases of young girls exhibiting early onset puberty from ingesting hormone-laced meat, dairy and eggs. Along those same lines, many people find themselves highly resistant to antibiotics while fighting an infection.

It's no wonder that consumers now prefer to purchase meat, chicken, dairy and eggs from organically raised, free-range, pasture-fed cows and organic, free-range, veggie-fed, hormone- and antibiotic-free hens. A whopping 80 percent of all antibiotics sold in the United States is used to raise chickens, pigs, cows and other livestock.[5]

"In the black, there is some white. In the wrong, there is some right. In the dark, there is some light. In the blind, there is some sight."

~ ABHINYANA

7

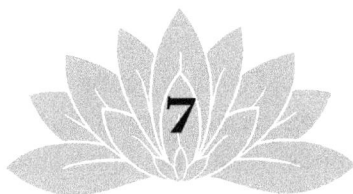

Back to Our Organic Roots

The developing technologies of industrialization took off like gangbusters, and there was little oversight by the FDA or USDA. Most unsuspecting consumers assumed that if it was manufactured, advertised and on the grocery store shelf, it must have gone through some kind of rigorous scrutiny regarding consumer safety. But that was *not* the case, and no one was the wiser.

Within time, the ever-adaptable general public became slowly lulled and oriented toward a diet based on convenience, availability and clever marketing. We were now consuming greater quantities of processed grain and flour products, refined sugar, factory-farmed animal meat and dairy products, imported fruits and veggies, and food items containing synthetic, chemicalized ingredients.

At the same time, a grassroots, natural-foods movement grew and continued to progress and propagate with great momentum. It monitored and scrutinized the many advances in modern technology, science, medicine and nutrition for safe consumption, and remained steadfast to the traditional ways and wisdom of living in harmony with nature.[6]

Fast-forward to the 21st century. Most of us have been exposed to the pros and cons of eating a contemporary diet, which includes commercially grown, packaged and chemically processed foods, versus the more naturally grown and processed, organic diet. We have a general idea of what *not* to eat, or at least what to cut down on. We have heard the conventional wisdom about moderating our sugar, alcohol, caffeine, meat, dairy, wheat and fat consumption. This begs the question: Well then, what's left?

I have found it easier and more effective to focus on what I *can* eat, rather than what I'm "not supposed" to. Instinctive eating is not about judging food as good or bad – or even being disciplined and controlled. It is about understanding how various stressors, foods, activity and weather can cause a sense of physical or emotional imbalance. It is also about choosing the most "corrective" food or activity to bring you back to center. Truth is, when you feel healthfully balanced, you can handle some of those processed "entertainment" foods much easier and with little downside of rocking the boat.

Instinctive Health is about developing an intuitive barometer that alerts you when your body, mind or emotions are out of sync. It's also about consciously choosing the most effective action or remedy to bring you back to center.

LIVING, EATING AND FEELING TUNED-IN

Is there a "perfect" way of eating? Nope, not in my opinion. There might be a particular food or meal that chimes you at any given time, but we mostly operate from a "what-am-I-in-the-mood-to-eat?" approach. The notion that there is one perfect diet for all people that when strictly adhered to, will afford health, happiness, and longevity is – sorry to say – a myth. How could there be a one-size-fits-all dietary plan? We all differ in genetics, culture, gender, age, health, environment and psychology. What *is* true is that we all essentially share the same genetic blueprint. What is also true is that our environment, lifestyle, activity level, attitude, relationships, and most of all, our diet, can and do influence that blueprint. This is what the original macrobiotic philosophy was based upon: harmonizing the *internal* environment of our body, mind and emotions, with the influences and circumstances of our *external* environment. That is also what this book is about: learning to develop an intuitive barometer that alerts you when your body or emotions get out of whack, and identifying the correct "adjustment" for nudging you back to center.

> "The root of all health is in the brain. The trunk of it is in emotion. The branches and leaves are the body. The flower of health blooms when all parts work together."
> – KURDISH PROVERB

I find for the most part, that living, eating and feeling tuned-in encourages a relaxed and responsive nature. It contributes toward an enjoyably healthy appetite, restful, rejuvenating sleep, a sharp, engaged mind, ample stamina, and an optimistic and considerate demeanor. And for those times when I feel off-kilter? I take note, catch it early and respond appropriately to correct the imbalance. I like having that knowledge *and* control. It is both reassuring and empowering.

The practice of eating and living in an instinctive manner has been around since the beginning of time. A tribe's survival was dependent upon it. Many nature-based healthful cultures and communities thrive today. Naturally there has been an evolutionary progression with each generation. A community's rhythm, pace, lifestyle and diet will always be influenced by its cultural and social mores, its location (mountain, sea, desert, plains) and its climate and growing season. Nothing is notably different or remarkable about the way tribe members live their lives, only that they have found a harmonious balance within nature, within their community, in their dietary customs and in their lifestyle that allows them to live long, healthy and contented lives.

By way of example, I want to introduce to you three communities. They all live instinctively and harmoniously within their culture and environment. They are all uniquely different in their climatic conditions, topography, growing seasons, personal philosophy, cultural traditions and attitude. Yet they all share similar health-promoting practices. They eat a predominantly plant-based (vegetarian) diet, do some sort of physical activity daily, have a strong sense of community and adhere to a spiritual practice or philosophy. These wholesome and healthful ways of living have been passed down for generations, and in many ways, mirror the holistic practices and lifestyles of today.

THE HUNZA PEOPLE

I first remember reading about the people living in the Hunza (pronounced Hoonza) Valley, located in the high mountain range of the Pakistani Himalayas, back in the 1970s. They were written about in an almost mythical way. They reportedly ate a mostly vegetarian diet with negligible amounts of meat and dairy, and lived well into their 90s and 100s. Not only did they live to a ripe old age, but they also seemed to flourish – with great enthusiasm, vigor and contentment. Recent websites and articles report they still do.

So what's their secret? No secret, it seems, but rather an ideally balanced blend of diet, lifestyle and attitude. The Hunzas diet consists primarily of freshly harvested seasonal fruits, leafy greens and root vegetables, grain, beans, raw unpasteurized milk and mineral-abundant glacial water. A large part of their diet is composed of whole grains, such as barley, millet, wheat and buckwheat. Whenever possible they sprout their beans and grain, making them more nutrient-filled and digestible. On a daily basis, they eat fruits and vegetables, both raw and steamed. The vegetables and fruits grown there include: potatoes, string beans, peas, carrots, turnip, squash, spinach, lettuce, apples, pears, peaches, apricots, cherries and blackberries. They also sun dry and store their fruit for use during the months when fruit is not as plentiful. No chemicals or artificial fertilizers of any kind are used in their gardens.

> *Organic meat, dairy, fruits and vegetables have been shown to have a more rich and robust flavor, and contain higher levels of antioxidant "life force" than commercially grown or processed foods.*

Meat is rarely eaten, mostly reserved for special occasions such as marriages and festivals. It is interesting to note that whenever meat is served, it is cut into small pieces, stewed for a long time, and the portions are very small, akin to a side dish. Chicken tends to be the most common source of animal protein, with the very occasional use of beef and mutton. Dairy plays an important part of their diet in the form of whole milk, butter, yogurt and cheese.

Along with their healthy diets, the Hunzas keep their bodies balanced and in shape by participating in everyday activities such as farming, animal care, construction, child-care, food-preparation, and their main means of transport – walking. For relaxation of mind and body, they have been known to practice various yoga techniques, such as slow, deep, rhythmic breathing, and take short meditation breaks throughout the day. This is not a whole lot different than the recommendations of many health practitioners today.

Not only is there a reported minimal amount of disease in this valley, but the Hunzas today appear to thrive. This can be attributed to their diet, attitude and lifestyle, but I also think it worthy to mention the practice of caloric-constraint. This is the idea of eating slower and more consciously – almost as a sacrament – along with consuming smaller portions. The combination is not meant to be – nor does it feel like a restriction. It is simply about eating in a conscious, more relaxed manner and stopping when you feel comfortably full. This practice of caloric-constraint is shared among all long-living, healthy people.

> *Caloric constraint is not about denying yourself by eating less; it's about eating in a more conscious and relaxed manner.*

I have personally experienced this way of eating, as well as its unconscious counterpart. Ever experience eating popcorn in a movie theater, and before you know it, you can feel the bottom of the bag? *Unconscious eating.* Or holiday meals, where you go back for seconds and thirds, ignoring that already-stuffed feeling? *Unconscious eating.* I have experienced both conscious and unconscious eating. My preferred way is the conscious practice of eating smaller portions, in a relaxed manner.

I have learned to eat my meals more "consciously" by doing a few simple things. I deliberately slow down my chewing, not unnaturally, but more as a reminding prompt. The great thing is that one prompt triggers the next. I then become aware of my breath. Again, nothing forced, but simply aware. I also focus on the flavor and enjoyment of the food I've got in my mouth. For me, the process is very similar to learning a new meditation – the more you do it, the more natural it becomes. And before you know it, the practice becomes automatically integrated, rather than something you have to remember to do.

Chewing well and slowly savoring your food makes it much easier to eat less without feeling deprived. The whole idea is to stop eating before you feel full. The brain starts registering feelings of fullness 10 to 20 minutes after we begin eating.

THE OKINAWAN PEOPLE

Much has been written about the tiny Japanese Island of Okinawa, located between mainland Japan and Taiwan. The number of Okinawans who reach 100 years of age is four to five times greater than that of Americans. If that's not impressive enough, they not only possess the biological markers of a much younger person, but their physical appearance, physical and mental agility, arterial function, bone density and hormone levels are those of someone much younger as well. Studies have also shown they have a notably lower rate of heart disease, stroke, obesity, cancer, dementia and other debilitating conditions, as compared with the levels we find in the United States.

As with other healthy, long-living cultures, the Okinawans' diet is primarily plant-based. Their diet includes a mixed array of vegetables with an emphasis on dark, leafy greens. They include a variety of fruits and berries, whole grains, especially brown rice, barley and millet, along with buckwheat noodles. They favor soybean products such as tempeh, miso, edamame, natto and small amounts of tofu. Various complementary seaweeds, herbs, spices, jasmine tea, plenty of water and small amounts of Omega-3-rich fish are also favored meal items. Lean meat, poultry and eggs are the occasional side dish, accounting for an approximate 3 percent of their overall diet. The Okinawans also enjoy a moderate inclusion of alcohol, with women averaging one drink a day and men averaging two.

They tend to consume much smaller amounts of sugar than most cultures. It is interesting to note that they rarely, if ever, consume dairy products yet have some of the lowest incidences of osteoporosis in the world. Once again, the practice of caloric-constraint comes into play with the Okinawans, who dine in a relatively relaxed manner until they are 80 percent full. This principle is called "hara hachi bu" and results in consuming 25 percent fewer calories than the average American consumes.[7]

"The more you eat, the less flavor; the less you eat, the more flavor."

– CHINESE PROVERB

Along with a nutrient-dense diet and smaller portions, the Okinawans' lifestyle and pace is low-stress compared to most. Rising at sunrise and following the rhythms of nature contributes to a more tranquil environment, pace and personal demeanor. Meditation is also an important aspect of keeping their daily outlook and attitude positive and peaceful. Last, there exists within the community a wonderful generosity of spirit, with a particular reverence and appreciation toward women and the elderly.

THE MONKS OF MT. ATHOS

Mt. Athos in Greece is considered the oldest surviving monastic community in the world. It has been the spiritual seat of Orthodox Christianity dating back to the Byzantine era, more than a thousand years ago.

As one might expect in a monastery setting, theirs is a chosen life of service and devotion to God, without the daily distractions of society. They have created an independent community that is resourcefully self-reliant and self-sustaining – one that has afforded the approximate 2,000 resident monks a remarkable level of health and vitality well into their advanced years.

According to research conducted on the monks' lifestyle and longevity, the single most important contributing factor in the low incidence of cancer is their vegetarian diet, rich in plant-based proteins and nutrients, with the occasional inclusion of fish. Research also indicates a surprising zero incidence of lung, bowel or bladder cancer among the monks, with an unusually low percentage of prostate cancer – four times less than the international average. The latter finding is even more extraordinary when you take into consideration that the monks participating in the study were between the ages of 50 and 104, when the incidence of prostate cancer is most prevalent. It was also reported that there were few, if any, reports or incidents of heart disease, cardiac arrest or stroke – and zero-incidence of Alzheimer's disease.

The monks' diet is similar to the Mediterranean diet so popularly written about today. The most notable difference in the monks' diet is that they consume little, if any, animal products. For more than half the year they are strictly vegan (no animal, dairy or egg products) and the rest of the time they are primarily vegetarian.

The health-promoting tenets of this monastic community are as follows:

- The monks never eat red meat and only sporadically eat fish.

- The bulk of their diet is whole grain, legumes, fruits, vegetables and herbs homegrown in each monastery's gardens and seasonally harvested.

- More than 200 days of the year – including all Mondays, Wednesdays, Fridays and religious holidays such as Lent and Advent – there are "abstention days," which are strictly vegan, with only one meal per day.

- All other days are considered non-fast days, during which dairy products, eggs, fish and home-brewed wine are moderately consumed if and when desired.

- Physical activity plays an important role throughout the monks' lives. This usually consists of maintaining the gardens and harvesting the produce; keeping the surrounding trees, brush and mountain trails cleared and trimmed back; and hauling any needed supplies along the mountain trails using pack mules.

- And last, but certainly not least, is the inspirational focus and foundation of their lives: the complete absorption of merging with God.[8]

The longevity these communities experience is remarkable, but what I find most inspiring is the dynamic health, physical agility, mental clarity and peaceful bearing they possess throughout their long lives, regardless of their differing locations, climates, landscape, growing seasons, lifestyles and cultural patterns. The research conducted on these varied communities bears out remarkably positive results. Each study shows that the combination of eating a nourishing, predominantly plant-based diet, partaking in physical activity, having a close, supportive social structure and fostering a kind, compassionate attitude toward all life promotes and maintains their healthful longevity. The diseases so prevalent in our own society today (heart ailments, cancer, arthritis, high blood pressure, diabetes, tuberculosis, hay fever, asthma, liver trouble, gall bladder trouble and constipation) are virtually nonexistent in these communities.

"Healing is a matter of time,
but it is also a matter of opportunity."
– HIPPOCRATES

Part Three
Principles for Cultivating an Instinctive Life

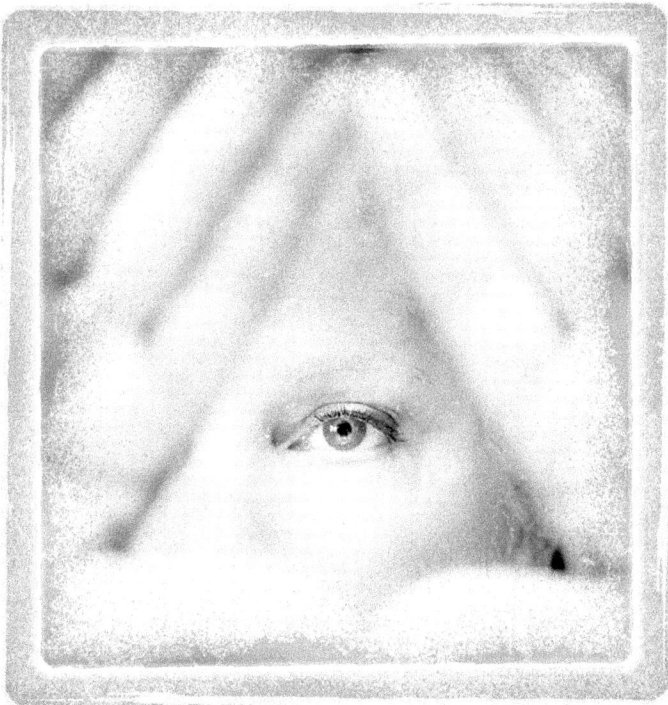

" *Life is a balance between rest and movement.* "

~ OSHO

8

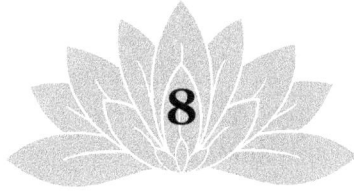

The Ancient Philosophy
of Balance

It's interesting to note the differences in how Eastern and Western medicine approach physical, mental and emotional health, function and regeneration.

Essentially, the Western model views the body more as a functioning machine with parts that are well designed, efficient and operational, become worn and need repairing, break down and need replacing. As long as the machinery functions within certain parameters, a person is considered reasonably healthy. Conventional Western medicine is allopathically oriented, meaning the focus is primarily concerned with treating the symptoms of an illness or disease, and repairing or replacing a malfunctioning part, usually with pharmaceuticals and surgery.

> "We don't have a healthcare system in this country, we have a disease-management system."
> - ANDREW WEIL, MD

The Eastern model views the body more as an energetic environment with frequently changing climatic conditions. These internal ecological patterns and conditions are compared to the environmental conditions within nature. There are climatic patterns, temperature variations, atmospheric pressure, aridness, thermal conditions and humidity levels. The Eastern perspective takes into consideration the body's entire "ecosystem" in determining the cause of the imbalance and uses different modalities including food, herbs, acupuncture and Qigong to activate, warm and nourish the body back into balance. The ultimate goal is to cultivate and support the bodily environment to be optimally self-functioning and self-regulating.

It is the Eastern model that I personally find so relatable and practical. Let's look at how this ancient philosophy of balance can be applied toward our own healthful enrichment.

The Eastern model came into being as a result of ancient Taoist scholars, healers and mystics developing a deeply insightful philosophical system that emphasized harmony between the body, mind and spirit, and the surrounding natural world. The philosophy was based on their observations, interactions and relationship with the unseen forces of nature. Through the application of this gathered wisdom, they were able to develop and deepen their physical vitality, mental clarity and spiritual awareness. It was believed that with determined focus and repetition, one could realize a transcendent state of physical and spiritual illumination.

"The ancient teaching of Tao tells us that knowing what
you really are is wisdom – and living it is virtue."
- ILCHI LEE

This profound philosophy of "energetic reciprocity" between spirit and matter was found to encompass the following principles:

- The all-encompassing Supreme Principle, called *The Tao* – a synonym for God.

- *Chi* – The creative energetic life force, permeating, "sparking" and animating all life within the Tao.

- The twofold, interactive and complementary expressions of *Yin and Yang* – The vibrational forces that are continually influencing, adjusting and transforming all aspects of life.

- The *Five Environmental Elements* or Energies within nature.

"The Tao is the One. From the One, comes Yin and Yang. From the two – Creative energy; From the Energy – ten thousand things, the forms of all creation. All Life embodies the Yin and embraces the Yang. Throughout their union, achieving harmony."
– TAO TE CHING, CHAPTER 42

The Tao (pronounced dow): The Absolute Guiding Principle – seen and unseen – within nature, our environment, our bodies and our minds, often described as The Way, The Path or The Principle – referring to "The Way of Nature," "The Path of Life" or "The Supreme Principle." The Tao is the all-encompassing source, the ultimate reality of existence, without shadowed interpretation. A synonym for God, it is the primordial force inhabiting and permeating all existence. It is likened to the Buddha Nature in Buddhism; Allah in Islam; God in Christianity;

and the Atman in Hinduism. In essence, the true Tao is an experiential state of complete Oneness.

> "In nature we never see anything isolated, but everything
> in connection with something else..."
> – GOETHE

Chi: The ever-present motivating *energetic life force* that permeates the earth, the atmosphere, the air we breathe, our physical body and the foods we eat. This same energetic life force is central to all philosophic traditions and is known by many different names. In Taoist or Chinese medicine, it is known as *Chi* or *Qi* (pronounced chee); in Japan, it's described as *Ki* (pronounced kee); in India, as *Prana* or *Shakti*; and in the West, it is referred to as *Life Force* or *Vitality*.

Yin and Yang Theory: (Yang is pronounced yong or yon) From within the Unity or single principle of Tao, emerge two vibrational forces, called Yin and Yang. These two complementary expressions of energy (Chi) are continuously flowing, animating, balancing, transforming and unifying all aspects of life and matter. Also known as the Theory of Opposing Principles, these two equally-powerful yet opposing forces manifest as feminine and masculine, darkness and light, interior and exterior, hidden and exposed, softness and hardness, cold and hot, and deficiency and excess. One force may be dominant in one moment and become its opposite in the next. Yin-Yang Theory is based on the continual adjustment and transformation of energy (Chi) within all aspects of our human experience and all natural phenomena.

The Five Environmental Elements or Energies: The Five Elements system is a comprehensive philosophy that categorizes all natural phenomena into five master groups or patterns in nature. The Five Environmental Energies are Wood, Fire, Earth, Metal and Water. Each of the Five Elements has correspondences with the seasons, with foods, flavors, bodily organs, senses, emotional states, activities and tendencies. The key to health and harmony is in understanding these correspondences and integrating them accordingly. This way, you're able to keep your internal environment balanced by taking conscious actions such as eating foods in season, being mindful of pace and portions, tuning in to body and emotions, engaging in activities that are nurturing, and adjusting to the changing world, circumstances and environment around you.

Adopt the rhythms of nature and
harmony will follow.

"*There is a life-force within your soul – seek that life.*"

~ Rumi

9

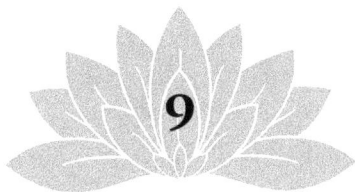

Chi: The Expression of Universal Energy

Let's take a look at how we begin to facilitate a feeling of connectedness and balance within our body, emotions and environment. A key factor is first understanding how to "assess and identify" various permutations of Chi (energy) flow and expression. We then "adjust and balance" that energy by using specific foods and activities – that will once again, provide a sense of equilibrium. The idea is to cultivate and circulate an abundance of "harmonizing" Chi that will support and sustain our optimal health and well-being. This philosophical and practical understanding of activating and engaging our innate brilliance to achieve ongoing balance, is the cornerstone of *Instinctive Health* and what I believe leads to a truly *Inspired Life*.

> *Instinctive Health is a process by which we "assess and identify" and "adjust and balance" the energy within our body, our life and our environment to achieve a harmonious state of health and well-being.*

In order to first assess the energetic tone and quality of Chi within our body and emotions, we need a conscious *qualifier* to identify these feelings. Often times we identify or recognize the emotional feeling of what we're experiencing, but we don't know how to describe or give language to it, especially a neutral, non-judgmental, descriptive type of language.

The way we learn to identify and describe a feeling within our body or emotions is similar to how we register and assign language to colors when describing a painting – kind of "temperature-based." For example, we've got the warm, autumnal colors such as gold, bronze, green, rust and yellow, which elicit a different feeling and response within us than the cooler colors of powder blue, turquoise, cobalt, violet and lavender. One color may elicit feelings of sunlit days and warm familiarity. The other may feel more spatial, cool, with reduced intensity. At different times and for different reasons, we may find ourselves drawn to one or the other. We often relate to people or environments in a similar way: "They have a very warm demeanor" or "The place felt cold somehow." Without being aware of it, we already assess, identify and describe our various experiences in a temperature-based way.

> "There is a voice that doesn't use words. Listen."
> – RUMI

Let's look at how we might apply a similar approach of interpreting, evaluating and communicating the various nuances of energetic manifestation within our bodies, behavior and environment. The concept of Chi allows us to do just that.

As mentioned before, within the traditional Taoist philosophy, there exists an ever-present motivating *energetic life force* that permeates the earth, the atmosphere, the air we breathe, our physical body, the foods we eat and all natural phenomena. This same energetic life force is central to all philosophic traditions and is known by many different names. We'll use the Taoist or Chinese medicine term Chi (chee) for our purposes when describing this life force energy.

> "Wisdom is to the soul what health is to the body."
> – CESAR VICHARD DE SAINT-REAL

Chi manifests as a dynamic presence or aliveness that can be seen, felt and experienced in virtually every aspect of life. This dynamic life force can range in vibration from the densest to the most refined, and can be readily observed in our physical bodies, personality, relationships, circumstances, environment and the foods we eat. When we say a person has good Chi, we mean that they come across as graceful, healthy, effective and usually quite charismatic. When organic fruits or vegetables are fresh and ripe, we would say that the Chi is at its prime – abundantly ideal in flavor, texture and nourishment. When an environment has good Chi flow, it feels embracing, enhancing and uplifting for us to be within that space. We could say that it wraps around us in a warm, inviting and comforting way. That is what Feng Shui is all about – good Chi flow.

When Chi is flowing cleanly, dynamically and effectively throughout the human body, it manifests as a robust energy and vitality that is visibly evident. When it is hampered, diminished or deficient in some way, we find the opposite, as if there is a kink in the life force hose.

> "Awareness is the greatest agent for change."
> – ECKHART TOLLE

Chinese medicine views the therapeutic qualities of Chi to operate in a three-fold manner: through (1) the food we eat; (2) the air we breathe; and (3) the rejuvenating, restorative and protective essence (Jing) generated within the body. We come into this world inheriting Jing from our parents, a genetic Chi of sorts, which gives us our initial foundation toward the development and maturation of all bodily processes – in essence, the root of our vitality.

In Chinese medicine, the kidney is viewed as the wellspring or source, where all vital energy or Chi is generated. It is also here that the reserves of Chi are stored, much like an energy bank, and accessible in times of need. It can fortify and assist in preventing illness, handling stress, healing existing maladies and sustaining health and longevity.

From the Western perspective of mechanics and function, the kidney is viewed as a filter or pump that removes waste products from the blood and regulates all fluid within the body – a very important and critical function. And, while the physical kidney certainly does perform that function, kidney Jing refers to a more subtle, refined and energetic quality.

How well we generate and utilize our personal Chi depends upon our physical constitution, belief systems, lifestyle, attitude, behavior, dietary habits, physical activity, time in nature and the climate in which we live. We could say that our good health and vitality are influenced and determined by the balance, strength and circulation of a refined and resilient Chi. Similarly, when that dynamic Chi (or energetic fire) becomes subdued, distorted or diminished, our immune system becomes compromised, making way for imbalances and illness to set in.

Personal Characteristics of Good, Strong Chi:

- Vital, energetic, dynamic
- Strength and endurance
- Responsive immune system
- Heals well, quickly, effectively
- Robust appetite and digestion
- Strong body, relaxed muscles, fluidity of movement
- Clarity of mind, good concentration
- Calm, receptive and considering demeanor
- Restful sleep

Personal Characteristics of Diminished, Deficient Chi:

- Lethargic, low energy
- Weakened, unresponsive immune system
- Reduced resistance, slow to heal
- Allergies, sensitivities, reoccurring illness or condition
- Depressed, self-absorbed, melancholic
- Sluggish, flaccid, overweight body
- Poor appetite and digestion
- Foggy brain, scattered concentration

> "When diet is wrong, medicine is of no use.
> When diet is correct, medicine is of no need."
> – ANCIENT AYURVEDIC PROVERB

To better understand how to use food as our medicine or balancing agent, let's look at the different ways Chi manifests within the plant and animal foods we consume – and why. The same way our personal Chi is affected by genetics, environment, nourishment, circumstances and the air we breathe, a similar comparison could be said for plant and animal species. The specificity of those conditions dictates the distinct characteristics, quality and strength of Chi within that particular group.

For example, if we look at an active fish, such as salmon, we would say it has a more dynamic Chi than say, an oyster, which leads a relatively dormant life by comparison.

A chicken that is allowed to move about freely (un-caged), dining on insects, has a cleaner, livelier Chi than a factory-farmed, caged hen.

You can imagine how organically raised animals that are allowed to roam freely (free-range), mature naturally and dine on pastured grass would have a more refined quality of Chi than animals that have been commercially-raised in crowded conditions with high levels of bacterial contamination, fed GMO grain, and are regularly inoculated with growth hormones and antibiotics.

In the plant kingdom, a vegetable like burdock root uses a strong, downward force to penetrate the hard soil in which it grows, and would therefore imbibe grounding and strengthening Chi. Compare that to a flowering vegetable such as broccoli, which grows upward and outward with a more blossoming, expansive energy. When considering the various properties of Chi, we are looking at the *energetic* qualities and influences that contribute toward that plant's growth, characteristics and formation – much like our human experiences contribute toward our character, fortitude and outward appearance. Does that vegetable grow quickly or take time? Is it sweet and juicy or bland and fibrous? Does it grow in harsh conditions or in a lush, fertile environment?

In my perception, whole foods in their natural state have a more powerful Chi than highly processed foods. Raw or "live" foods have a different *vibrancy* of Chi than, say, cooked foods. Again, it's the energetic "tone" or quality of a food – that which gives it its specific characteristics that we're looking for. This is why, for example, when I'm shopping for produce I will look for well-formed, brightly colored vegetables and fruits that emanate a vibrant, robust quality – similar to the energy I sense in well-balanced, healthy people.

Given my prior raw food philosophy, I had believed that when food was cooked, the heat destroyed much of its nutrients. As I grew in understanding, I realized there were many different ways that energy or Chi flow can be diluted, altered, enhanced or transferred into our food, body or environment.

I also experienced how the energetic properties within food can be improved or specifically influenced by using different methods of preparation, serving, storage and cooking:

- *Preparation/Serving methods* (cold, hot, salty, sweet, bland, seasoned)

- *Storage methods* (refrigerated, frozen, canned, dried, fermented)

- *Cooking methods* (sautéing, steaming, baking, pressure-cooking)

Armed with this new shift in perception, I was able to view the fire, or "energetic" heat within my cooked food, as being transferred or imbibed into me in a positive and enhancing way.

> "Intelligence is the ability to adapt to change."
> – STEPHEN HAWKING

Understanding the principle of Chi and how it flows, moves and expresses itself was incredibly liberating for me. With the ability to "assess and identify" and "adjust and balance" the energetic qualities, strengths and differentiations of Chi, I could now create the qualities and results I desired. I felt like I had been gifted a magic power that allowed me to direct and utilize this wonderfully multi-faceted energy toward my highest good. Yin-Yang Theory will further demonstrate how we can create balance with the process of energy exchange.

10

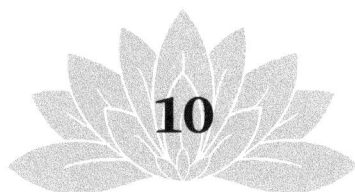

The Harmonizing Expression of Yin and Yang

Within nature, the principles of Yin and Yang are used to further describe the breakdown of Chi energy that permeates and governs all life. Yin is the *outward* spinning, loosening force creating expansion, diffusion, lightness, slower motion and lower, cooler temperatures. Yang is the *inward* spinning, tightening force creating contraction, density, heaviness, rapid motion and higher, hotter temperatures. Each force's movement, expression and tendency are dependent upon the law of relativity and relationship – that everything is relative to something else. Everything in nature has its complementary opposite, be it a physical characteristic or an emotional one that brings it into balance or wholeness. Yin and Yang are not fixed conditions, but rather energetic tendencies that continuously cycle, flow and interact. Day turns into night, winter flows into spring, heat cools down, moisture dries up, undeveloped becomes ripe and activity eventually rests. I like to think of Yin and Yang as the dual "personalities" of Chi, with each having a different disposition, behavior, quality, momentum, temperature and charm.

In looking at the Taoist Yin-Yang symbol, we have the circle representing the One, the Tao – and within the Tao we have the two complementary expressions of Chi, manifesting as Yin and Yang energy. In each of these individual energies, whether separate or blended, there is the opposite colored dot in each, representing the interdependence and inseparableness of each aspect's properties, influences and nuances within the other. These two energies are in a continual dance – interacting, blending and flowing within and throughout all natural phenomena.

Yin	*Yin-Yang*	*Yang*

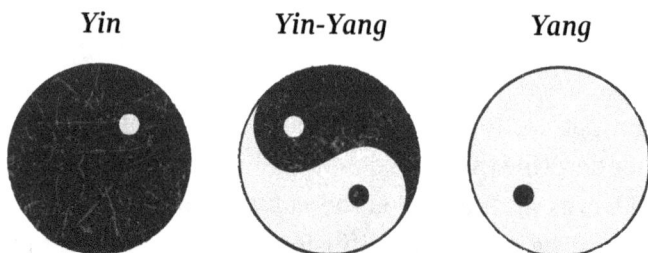

The Taoist Yin-Yang symbol embodies the harmonious merging of both individual energies.

The literal translation of Yin is *shadow* – symbolized by the dark circle – and is said to represent "the shady side of a mountain." The literal translation of Yang is *light*, and represents the illumined or sunny side of the mountain – and is signified by the light circle. Consequently, daytime (light) would be considered Yang, while nighttime (dark) is considered Yin. When we think of winter, we can imagine the distinct qualities of coldness, darkness, dampness, inwardness, stillness and potential (gestation of ideas), all of which register as Yin qualities. When we think of summer, the qualities are hotness, brightness, dryness, outward activity and manifestation (making things happen), all of which register as Yang qualities.

Using the analogy of Yin and Yang representing the two *personalities* of Chi, we observe the contrasting, yet complementary qualities of feminine and masculine, intuitive and logical, softness and hardness, hidden and exposed, night and day, cold and hot, moistness and dryness, and loosening and tightening.

Of these two energies, the Yin feminine principle is considered the softer, quieter, relaxed, more receptive energy. Much like we feel when we're surrounded by nature, in the presence of a beloved, beholding a magnificent vista, or completely absorbed in meditation. We feel *positively* vulnerable, *invitingly* receptive and *effortlessly* attuned. We classify this feeling and energy as Yin. Yin is described as the flowing, or less dynamic energy (relative to Yang) that promotes reflection, relaxation and creativity. Yin energy is easy and fluid, much like water. Generally considered to be more expanded, ethereal and soft – and in its most esoteric form it is considered dormant or hidden away. When the Yin aspect of our behavior manifests in a balanced and healthy manner, we find ourselves feeling calm, open-minded, intuitive, imaginative, creative, harmonious, peaceful, sympathetic, sensitive, patient and cooperative. Even in simply imagining these qualities, we are easily transported to that state of mind. Most of us strive to live in this harmoniously balanced place as often as possible.

Much like nature, our circumstances in life are never permanent – but fluid and changeable.

Yang energy is described as the active or more dynamic principle, stimulating movement, progress and activity. Yang is the energy that quickens, animates and enlivens – much like we feel when we're passionately drawn or compelled toward a person or place, or when we assume a more driven or dominant role in a relationship, a work project, or physical adventure. It is the dynamic energy of feeling confident, motivated and compelled to actively "move toward." In its extreme form, Yang energy can have an accelerated, pressured or even explosive quality. When we are healthy and balanced in our Yang behavior, we find ourselves feeling positive, grounded, confident, passionate, assertive, independent, focused, ambitious, enthusiastic and effective. You can see how these Yang qualities would be more desirable in our urban, production-oriented culture. These qualities speak to the passionate, capable, independent and productive side of us.

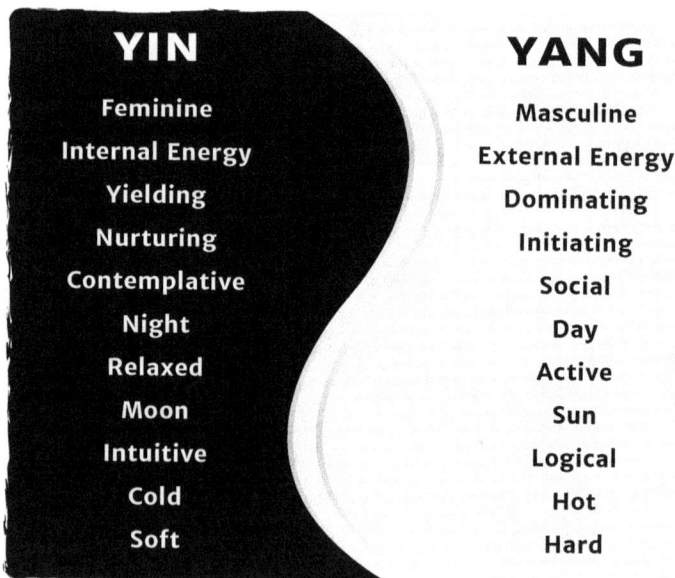

YIN	YANG
Feminine	Masculine
Internal Energy	External Energy
Yielding	Dominating
Nurturing	Initiating
Contemplative	Social
Night	Day
Relaxed	Active
Moon	Sun
Intuitive	Logical
Cold	Hot
Soft	Hard

Our mental, physical and emotional behavior will often times overlap and blend each energy into the other. For example, we may feel confident and assured in one moment, and unsure and off-kilter in the next. We may feel social and outgoing one day, and quiet and laidback the next. We may feel elated, and then find ourselves melancholy; feeling relaxed and easy, then uptight and anxious. You get the picture. Yin and Yang qualities manifest in degrees, nuances and gradations, and are always relative to something else. Nothing in the natural world is ever exclusively Yin or Yang. We can use the energetic qualities of Yin and Yang to identify and communicate how we are feeling physically, mentally and emotionally.

Let's look at why and how being able to "assess and identify" and "adjust and balance" the different *personalities* or energetic expressions of Yin and Yang would be helpful.

IT IS ALL ABOUT BALANCE

When we look at the complementary ways nature balances itself, we observe that the local foods growing in a hot, tropical Yang climate tend to have the effectively balancing Yin properties of moistening, refreshing and cooling down the body. This is precisely what the juicy, sweet, tropical fruits such as citrus, papaya, mango, pineapple, melons and coconuts, do for us. And let's not forget the refreshing, succulent vegetables, such as summer squashes, cucumbers, tomatoes, spinach, eggplants, leafy lettuces and bell peppers.

> "Happiness is not a matter of intensity but of balance,
> order, rhythm and harmony."
> – THOMAS MERTON

Typically, this type of climate also promotes a more physical and activity-driven lifestyle, resulting in a more dynamically "heated" body. Think beach environment. If you have ever lived or vacationed in places such as Jamaica, Hawaii or

Mexico, you know what I mean. You're on a hot sunny beach and maybe you have walked, jogged, hiked and been active for many hours. You're in a Yang environment and these are typical Yang activities. Your body is quite heated and you may be feeling dehydrated. What sounds perfect in this moment? How about having a cold swim, a cold drink and relaxing in a cooler environment. Once the body cools down, the mind follows suit by relaxing and slowing down, often ending up in a catnap. These are all considered Yin qualities or attributes.

For most of us, there is an instinctive tendency to have Yin, cooling foods in the hot summer and Yang, warming foods in the cold winter. Much like my winter experience in Mt. Shasta, we're naturally drawn to hot, salty soups, flavorful satisfying meals and heated, warming beverages in colder weather.

So, what are the properties that make a particular food more Yang and therefore more grounding? The answer is *time, heat* and *salt*. Let's look at why.

Time: Foods that take longer to grow, longer to cook and longer to digest, all generate more heat in the body. Heat always registers as a more Yang energy.

Let's use meat as an example. In this case, we'll use a cow. It takes many months for a cow to grow to maturity, cooking time for meat is considerably longer than plant-based foods and actual digestion time for meat takes a good few hours. Meat is, therefore, considered one of the most energetically Yang foods we could eat, especially when compared to plant foods.

An example of a more Yang vegetable would be winter squash. It takes longer to grow, longer to cook and longer to digest, therefore producing more heat than, say, a fast-growing, watery summer squash. Summer squashes grow in a hot climate and are meant to cool you down. They grow, cook and digest faster relative to winter squash, and thereby promote a cooling, moistening effect on the body.

Heat: This is the easiest and most obvious quality to understand. Adding heat or fire of any kind produces a warmer temperature and energy in the body. Think of a hot bowl of soup. Think of soaking in a hot Epsom-salts bath. The element of fire also registers in the body as an energetic force, with its own qualities and attributes. The most Yang method of cooking would be baking, as it is hot, dry and involves time, all Yang attributes.

Salt: Salt has a contracting (drawing in) and grounding quality. It tends to make things shrink or shrivel. Think of a juicy cucumber. If it sits in salt brine over time, it becomes a contracted version of itself – a pickle. Pickles are considered a Yang food because they contain both the qualities of time (aged/fermented) and salt. Aged, salted, hard cheeses would also be more Yang than, say, softer, sweeter and minimally aged cheeses.

> *The contributing properties that make a particular food more Yang and therefore more grounding, are time, heat and salt.*

You would naturally be attracted to the heating and drying influence of a more Yang-oriented diet if you were displaying Yin watery symptoms, such as bloating, allergies, runny nose, congestion and cold hands and feet. If you were experiencing Yin watery symptoms on an emotional level, you would most likely be inclined toward feeling overly-sensitive, "not-quite-right" in your body and welling up and teary – doesn't matter if the tears are happy or sad ones. It is simply the body's way of eliminating the excess Yin fluid to balance itself.

In contrast, if your body is experiencing excess Yang symptoms, such as feeling overheated, parched, restless, tense and agitated, then a more Yin diet would be appropriate. In such a case, the emotional display would be one of reaction and impatience – much like a pressure cooker releasing excess heat and pressure. The recommended Yin-leaning diet would consist of fresher, lighter, plant-based foods: raw fruit and veggie salads, avocado, nuts, seeds, lightly steamed vegetables, rice, quinoa and small amounts of lean protein. These balancing foods would have the desired effect of moistening, refreshing and cooling down the "heated" Yang body.

YIN AND YANG PROPERTIES OF FOOD

Foods are classified according to:

- The rapidity of growth – fast or slow
- The direction in which it grows – above the ground or below
- The climatic environment where food is grown – temperate or tropical
- A food's flavor, sweetness, saltiness and texture
- A food's temperature and preparation method
- A food's physical and psychological effect on the body and mind

Characteristics of Yin Food:*
(cooling, moistening, refreshing)

- Grows in warmer climates
- Grows fast, grows above ground (think lettuces, tomatoes)
- Sweet, tender and juicy
- Perishes quickly (think leafy greens, salad makings, sprouts)
- Quickly digests
- Raw, refrigerated or frozen
- Faster cooking time
- Chemically processed (extreme Yin)
- Leaves of a plant, fruits of a tree
- Spicy, aromatic oils and fats

* Eating a balanced-diet of Yin foods will help us to feel relaxed, easy, open, intuitive, creative, compassionate, contented and peaceful.

Characteristics of Yang Food:*
(warming, drying, grounding)

- Grows in cooler climates
- Grows slower, below ground
- Salty, tough and fibrous
- Keeps and stores well
- Longer digestion time
- Cooked, hot or room temperature
- Slower cooking time
- Aged, pickled, dried
- Stems, roots and seeds of a plant
- Bland, dense and dry

* Eating a balanced-diet of Yang foods will help us to feel energetic, grounded, competent, self-assured, focused, quick-witted, ambitious and motivated.

A BALANCED BASELINE DIET

As we've established, a healthy, healing and regenerating body is the likely result of applying the energetic principles of Yin and Yang to our daily diet and lifestyle. It is the most predictable way to bring any particular disparity, condition or symptom into balance. For most of us, we tend to feel and do better with a slightly Yang-leaning diet, which offers a more stable and consistent feeling within our body and mind. That's because Yang energy moves downward and inward within the body, affecting a more even-keeled, *centered* feeling. Such a diet might include foods like lean animal protein, eggs, cooked grains, beans, root veggies, winter squashes, leafy greens, sea vegetables, pickled/ fermented foods and maybe some salty whole-grain crackers and chips. If we were to describe the mental or emotional quality that Yang foods provide, it would be more "steady-eddy," grounded and focused – with a confident sense of self. You can see why, in our Western "power and productivity" oriented lifestyles, it is quite advantageous to foster a more Yang energy than Yin. In other words, we're much more *effective* at work when we're sociably affable verses reserved; physically strong verses fragile; proficient more than incapable; and more self-assured than timid.

> "No disease that can be treated by diet should be treated with any other means."
> – MAIMONIDES

When we look at Nature's infinite wisdom, we notice that the foods that grow naturally in a four-season or higher-elevation climate tend to be the more slow burning, warming foods – best suited for fluctuating temperatures. This type of climate also tends to promote a mellower pace and demeanor within its populace. This is especially so in the slower, quieter, winter months, when we're much less active. We also find ourselves feeling more internal and introspective during these times. We crave hot baths and warm fires, we're more inclined to cozy-down with a good book, and we typically go to bed earlier and sleep a bit longer.

Food wise, we are naturally drawn to a more substantial, savory, heat-generating kind of diet during the cooler months. Included in that list are hot soups and stews, hearty grains, casseroles, winter squashes and warmth-producing seasonings such as cayenne, cinnamon, ginger, black pepper, garlic and onion. Many folks are drawn to animal products, which makes perfect sense because they are very warming.

On the other hand, if you happen to reside in a tropical climate or are simply vacationing during the warmer summer months, you would most likely find yourself drawn to eating a lighter, more cooling, Yin oriented diet. Lots of cool beverages, fresh seasonal fruit and vegetables, salads, guacamole, salsa, and maybe some fish and margaritas would be in order. These would all have the refreshing effect of cooling down the body – especially if you were doing any kind of physical activity.

Below, you'll find a good example of a wholesome, baseline-diet with foods that make up a balanced core of your diet, while you choose complementary Yin- or Yang-leaning foods, as needed or desired. Those might include alcohol, sweets, desserts on the Yin side – and meat, fowl, fish or salty, fermented/aged foods on the Yang side.

In looking at the Energetic Food Values chart, we see the various gradations of extreme Yin substances on the bottom left, all the way around the pyramid towards the most Yang foods on the bottom right. We observe that all foods are relative to one another on the energetic-spectrum.

You will find yourself continually adjusting your diet accordingly – depending upon your physical, mental, emotional and environmental condition.

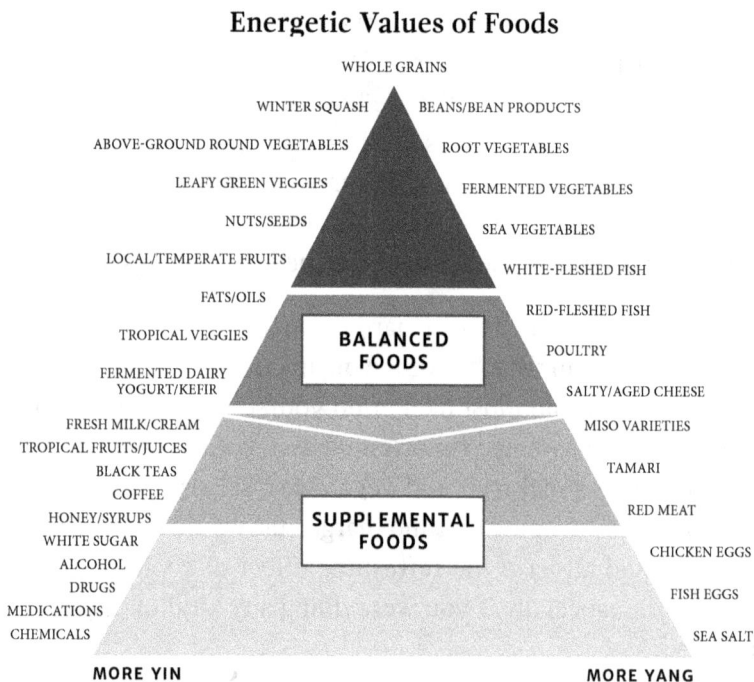

Energetic Values of Foods

WHOLE GRAINS

WINTER SQUASH   BEANS/BEAN PRODUCTS

ABOVE-GROUND ROUND VEGETABLES   ROOT VEGETABLES

LEAFY GREEN VEGGIES   FERMENTED VEGETABLES

NUTS/SEEDS   SEA VEGETABLES

LOCAL/TEMPERATE FRUITS   WHITE-FLESHED FISH

FATS/OILS   RED-FLESHED FISH

TROPICAL VEGGIES   **BALANCED FOODS**   POULTRY

FERMENTED DAIRY YOGURT/KEFIR   SALTY/AGED CHEESE

FRESH MILK/CREAM   MISO VARIETIES

TROPICAL FRUITS/JUICES

BLACK TEAS   TAMARI

COFFEE

HONEY/SYRUPS   **SUPPLEMENTAL FOODS**   RED MEAT

WHITE SUGAR   CHICKEN EGGS

ALCOHOL

DRUGS   FISH EGGS

MEDICATIONS

CHEMICALS   SEA SALT

MORE YIN   **MORE YANG**

BASELINE DIET OF NATURAL FOODS
(Organic, when possible)

> "Organic farming provides the surest path to improved nutritional quality in our widely consumed fruits and vegetables. Vine ripened organic produce tastes better and produces more nutrients per calorie consumed."
> – CHARLES BENBROOK, PH.D.

Whole Grains:
(All low gluten or gluten-free)

- Brown, red or black rice
- Brown Basmati rice
- Quinoa (pronounced keen-wah)
- Millet
- Buckwheat
- Rolled oats
- Spelt
- Wild rice
- Blue corn/yellow corn

The most nutritious way to consume grain is in its whole, unrefined form – with the outer bran layer and the inner germ still intact.

Root vegetables: carrot, beet, fennel, garlic, ginger, jicama, onion, parsnip, radish, shallot, sweet potato and yam.

Winter squashes: acorn, butternut, Delicata, Hokkaido, Hubbard, Kabocha, pumpkin and spaghetti squash.

Seasonal green and low-starch vegetables: asparagus, basil, bok choy, broccoli, brussels sprouts, cabbage, cauliflower, chard, collards, kale, green beans, summer squash and spinach.

Salad fixings: arugula, avocado, carrot, celery, cilantro, cucumber, mixed lettuces, parsley, daikon, radish, baby spinach, scallion and mixed sprouts.

Veggie-sourced protein:*

- Baked firm tofu (3 oz. = 14 grams)
- Tempeh (3 oz. = 12 grams)
- Lentils (1/2 cup = 9 grams)
- Edamame 1/2 cup = 8 grams)
- Black beans (1/2 cup = 8 grams)
- Garbanzos/Chickpeas (1/2 cup = 7 grams)
- Quinoa (1 cup = 8 grams)
- Almonds (1/4 cup = 8 grams)
- Pumpkin seeds (1/4 cup = 9 grams)
- Sunflower seeds (1/4 cup = 6 grams)
- Sesame seeds (raw tahini) (2 Tbsp. = 8 grams)
- Hempseed (1 Tbsp. = 5 grams)
- Mixed bean and seed sprouts (sprouting increases protein availability by 30 percent)

* *Protein amounts vary by brand and processing.*

Animal protein: any organic, free-range, pasture-fed meat, organic, free-range chicken and eggs, and fresh, wild caught fish.

Dairy: The word *judicious* comes to mind when consuming dairy products. However, if like most, you find yourself craving an occasional bit of cheese, then it's best to have the older, drier and saltier cheeses, such as aged Cheddar, dry Jack, Parmigiano Reggiano, Swiss Emmental and Gruyere. They are considerably more Yang (aged and salty), and tend to be less mucus forming. Fermented dairy products, such as yogurt, kefir, sour cream and cultured butter, also seem to do well in most bodies when eaten in moderation.

Seeds: pumpkin seeds, sunflower seeds, sesame seeds (raw tahini), hemp seeds and chia seeds.

Nuts: almonds, walnuts, hazelnuts, pecans and pine nuts.

Hearty, warming soups: miso soup, Thai Tom Yum (lemongrass, cilantro, chili oil, garlic), leafy greens and root vegetable soup, or organic chicken/meat broth soups.

> *My favorite nutritious plant-based foods include: Legumes: tempeh, lentils, edamame, baked tofu and various bean-hummus, as well as nuts: almonds, hazelnuts and walnuts. Favored seeds include: pumpkin seeds, sunflower seeds, sesame tahini; and preferred grains: quinoa and brown rice. The veggies I favor are: broccoli, kale, chard, collards and cilantro.*

Wholegrain breads, cereals and crackers: Gluten-free, brown rice bread or muffins; organic, fruit-sweetened cereals, whole-grain granolas, rolled oats or cooked brown-rice cereal; sprouted-grain, Manna, Essene or Ezekiel breads and wholegrain crackers; quality gluten-free products are now available using brown rice, coconut, blanched almond, hazelnut, buckwheat and tapioca flours.

Cooked/roasted sea vegetables: Arame: (calcium), Hijiki: (calcium), Nori: (protein), Kombu and Wakame: (calcium) and Dulse: (iron). Mineral-rich and balancing for both male and female hormones.

> *Seaweeds are highly nutritious. They are rich in minerals and nutrients essential for balancing hormones and metabolism, reducing stress and fatigue, nourishing bone, hair and nails, and enhancing a healthy glowing complexion. They're also helpful in expelling heavy metals and radioactive substances from the body.*

Warming herbs: cinnamon, garlic, ginger, turmeric, black pepper, cayenne pepper and chili powder.

Seasonal fruits: apples, apricots, berries, cherries, figs, melons, nectarines, peaches, pears and plums.

Natural fats: avocado, olives, cold-pressed, unrefined, virgin oils (coconut, olive, sesame, walnut, flax, hemp, avocado) and organic butter.

Fermented foods: Kim chi, tempeh, sauerkraut, natural pickles, kombucha tea, beer, yogurt, kefir and miso paste. Fermented foods are highly beneficial as they help fortify the intestinal flora with health-promoting probiotics. These healthy bacteria assist with digestion, absorption and in maintaining a strong, responsive immune system.

Fermented foods promote beneficial probiotic gut-bacteria, improve digestion, increase immunity and enhance nutrient absorption – resulting in a healthier, stronger body and immune system.

Natural sweeteners: organic maple syrup, brown rice syrup, yacon syrup, Jerusalem artichoke syrup, coconut sugar, stevia, raw, dark agave and local honey.

A few personal tips:

- *I find the most balanced soy products to use regularly are organic tempeh, miso, tamari (all fermented), baked-tofu (firm) and edamame (fresh soy bean pods).* I find them easier to digest and their nutrients more available – as compared with the highly processed soy products such as soy cheese, soy-meat, textured soy-protein and soy ice cream. Best to eat these kinds of processed soy products only on occasion. For those who prefer dairy but are lactose intolerant (not producing the needed enzyme to digest dairy sugar), there are organic companies (Green Valley Organics), which offer lactose-free yogurt and kefir. A lactase-enzyme is added to break down the milk sugar.

- *Whenever buying cheese, preferably organic – I check to see if rennet is listed on the label.* Animal rennet traditionally comes from the lining of a calf's stomach, and as a vegetarian, I would always prefer the microbial enzymes to the animal rennet. Enzymes are used during the cheese-making process to separate the milk curds (solids) from the whey (liquid).

- *Regarding commercial dairy products typically laced with antibiotics and hormones – it's always best to go with organic products when that option is available.* However, there are some good, natural dairy farms that have not been officially "certified-organic" and would not there-fore, bear such a label. Nonetheless, they *are* labeled as antibiotic-free and rBGH-free. rBGH (recombinant Bovine Growth Hormone) is a controversial genetically engineered synthetic hormone injected into cows to increase milk production. These hormones have an extremely debilitating effect on the cow's health, which in turn affects the quality and safety of the milk produced.

- *When making miso soup, the salty, dark misos are recommended in the winter.* The lighter miso's (white and yellow) are sweeter, less salty, less fermented and are better suited for the spring and summer. Since miso contains living enzymes, it's best not to let the soup come to a boil, as boiling destroys the beneficial enzymes and nutrients. The easiest way to avoid this is to make the soup first and add miso right before serving. When reheating, use a low-heat setting.

- *Short grain brown rice is best used in the cooler, winter months, as it burns slower and produces more heat in the body.* The reason it burns slower is due to its more glutinous nature. The same would go for sweet rice (japonica) used in making "mochi" (rice cake or rice confection). Long grain brown rice is more balancing and better suited for the warmer months.

Noteworthy Condiments:

- **Tamari, shoyu, miso:** Traditional tamari, shoyu and miso are all naturally aged and fermented, organic soybean seasonings that contain many medicinal and nutritional properties. Unlike shoyu, tamari does not contain wheat and is an excellent seasoning for those who prefer a wheat-free diet. The typical amount of time that tamari is aged or fermented is between six months and two years. It contains living enzymes that help with our digestion and are assistive in strengthening the immune system. Beware of "hydrolyzed" soy sauces processed with caramel coloring and alcohol. Companies use these ingredients in lieu of naturally fermenting the soybeans.

- **Himalayan crystal salt:** Ones of the reasons this particular salt is considered so beneficial to us is that the same 84 natural minerals and elements found in the body are also contained in Himalayan salt. It's also because these ancient sea salt beds have remained covered for more than 200 million years by a protective layer of lava, and there's been zero exposure to toxins and impurities. Especially when compared to the different varieties of sea salt that have been exposed to industrial, atmospheric, radioactive and chemical pollutants, Himalayan salt is believed to be the purest form of salt found on earth. The inherent minerals are in a colloidal form, allowing for the most effective absorption and bio-energetic utilization.

- **Coconut oil:** Organic, cold-pressed virgin coconut oil is preferred. It is an excellent and healthy saturated fat for cooking and sautéing, because it's not affected by high heat. Lauric acid, capric acid and caprylic acid are all beneficial fatty acids found in coconut oil, and are known to have antimicrobial, antioxidant, antifungal and antibacterial properties. Coconut oil also makes a wonderfully effective moisturizing preventative for dry, aging or flakey skin when used topically.

- **Sweeteners:** Barley malt, brown-rice syrup, ground sugar cane (Sucanat, "sugar cane natural"), coconut palm sugar and syrup, Yacon (Peruvian tuber), Jerusalem Artichoke syrup, raw, dark Agave, (avoid highly processed agave), date sugar and paste, maple syrup and fruit juice concentrates from apples, pears or grapes. Preferably organic. Soaking organic raisins or goji berries in water, and using the juice, also provides a mildly flavored sweetener.

- **Vinegars:** Vinegar, like any fermented food, helps stimulate our digestive juices, such as hydrochloric acid in the stomach, which in turn, aids with digestion. (Apple cider, brown rice, balsamic, umeboshi plum, Saba vinegars).

11

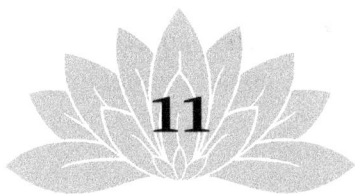

Identifying Yin and Yang Imbalances Within the Body

Ideally, what we're shooting for when we discuss imbalances is that perfect equilibrium of feeling good, solid and easy within our physical body, so that we can move through life effectively and efficiently. When the first signs of an imbalance show up, we need to take heed. We then identify whether the symptoms are Yin or Yang and utilize the most counterbalancing remedy. Classic Yin symptoms are distinct and noticeable, with watery indicators such as allergies, sneezing, congestion, runny nose and bloating. And typically our body temperature has cooled down to the point of feeling chilled.

The physical or bodily symptoms of being "Too Yin" (cool, damp and watery) are listed below. If you are aware of these "damp" symptoms or patterns in your body, you would need to counterbalance by adding some heating and drying foods, using warmth-producing cooking methods and engaging in some type of warming activity. It's essential to create enough heat to "steam out", dry out or otherwise absorb the excess fluid or dampness in the body. You would also want to avoid (or reduce) any refrigerated, cold or iced food or beverages, and avoid exposure to colder temperatures.

Overly Yin Symptoms:
(Damp patterns or conditions)

- Moist conditions (runny nose, loose bowels, abundant mucus, phlegm, yeast infections)
- Tendency to feel cool or chilled in body
- Cold hands and feet
- Stuffy nose, postnasal drip, sinus headache
- Preference for warm food and beverage
- Retention of fluids, bloated
- Tendency to dress warmly, drawn to heated environments
- Pale complexion, lack of color and energy
- Tendency to feel drained and tired. Wanting to sleep
- Minimal appetite or thirst
- Mentally sluggish, foggy-headed
- Dull, lingering aches and pains
- Shortness of breath. Difficulty inhaling deeply
- Muscles are soft, fleshy and weak
- Slower metabolism
- Symptoms, aches and pains, worsen in damp or cold weather
- Feeling depressed, resigned, worried or withdrawn

ADDRESSING IMBALANCED YIN SYMPTOMS

In this category, we are talking about the energetic properties of Yin foods and why they affect us the way they do. We are mostly concerned with why and how these particular foods throw us out of whack. It's not about a certain food, drink or substance being "bad" for you – but rather the energetic influence of any food, substance or activity acting as a therapeutic curative or aggravator.

In establishing how to address Yin symptoms in the body, we'll also look at the various gradations with which to identify foods in the Yin category. Keep in mind, that all foods are relative to one another on either side of the energetic-spectrum. We note that fruits are typically more Yin than veggies; veggies more Yin than grains; and grains more Yin than meat. However, there's a further breakdown or classification within each food group. For example, summer squash (sweeter, juicier, faster-growing) is considered more Yin than winter squash. Tropical fruits are more Yin than temperate fruit. Papaya is more Yin than apple.

Yin foods have a cooling, moistening effect on the body, and typically grow in warmer climates. They tend to grow fast, above the ground and are prone to perish quickly. Think of lettuces, cucumbers, tomatoes and melons. Yin foods are also known to digest quickly. They are mostly served raw, refrigerated and iced – as in salads, chilled foods, juices and cold drinks.

It's not about a certain food, drink or substance being "bad" for you. It's about the energetic understanding that anything can have an invigorating or debilitating effect on the body.

Processed foods such as white sugar, candy, ice cream, sodas, flavored syrups, diet-foods and chemical additives all fall into the "extreme" Yin category, due to their concentrated sugar and resulting impact on our body's chemistry. Taken in moderation, we're generally OK. Taken in excess, watch out. Think kids, the day after Halloween. Off. The. Wall.

Alcohol and marijuana also fall into this concentrated or extreme Yin category because of the altering impact and influence (expansive, relaxing) on our body, mind and emotions. An alcoholic drink or two (depending on the person) can be "good medicine" after a heated, stress-filled day or week. However, if you're already exhibiting Yin symptoms physically and emotionally, and you choose to have a drink or two, this will typically exacerbate the "existing" Yin imbalance.

So, what actually makes a particular food or substance fall into the "extreme" Yin category? Extreme Yin foods are those that initially give us some kind of blood sugar boost or "rush" and are accompanied afterwards by a downward-spiraling, low blood sugar "crash." This could be a head rush from alcohol, a sugar rush from sweets or a body rush from caffeine. Regardless of the cause, the body registers an infusion of sugar – otherwise known as a sugar glut or overload.

> *Extreme Yin foods initially give us a desirable boost or rush. A head rush from alcohol, a sugar rush from sweets or a body rush from caffeine. In each case, the body registers a sugar glut. The challenge is how to handle the accompanying sugar-crash afterwards.*

Imagine for a moment, if you will, that for a solid week, you ate and drank one or all of the following foods and nothing else. This would essentially include a seven-day fast of coffee, ice cream, soda, candy, beer and wine only. You might initially feel okay with the coffee pumping you up, the sweet tasting treats satisfying you, and the alcohol relaxing you. You might even be able to last a couple days eating this way, but after that, it's guaranteed that you'd feel out of whack. That's because, these kinds of ancillary foods are not considered "real" food. We're talking wholesome, nourishing, naturally grown food that supplies the body and mind with fortifying sustenance.

Let's break it down. In the case of alcohol, it may initially feel warm or hot going down (seemingly Yang), but soon enough, we feel a "heady" expanded effect and our mood becomes more relaxed – both considered Yin symptoms. Again, a little bit is generally fine, but over do it and the body is thrown into the "extreme" Yin category.

An example might be where you're already experiencing Yin symptoms in your body – feeling "on the verge" of a cold or flu – and you go have a few drinks with friends. There's a very good chance that the energetically-Yin alcohol will have you experiencing a full-blown cold by morning. Or, how about you've got the same conditions, and you find yourself on an airline flight for many hours inside the chilled compartment with recirculating air? These are perfect conditions to aggravate your already compromised immunity.

Now, you might be wondering why coffee is in this Yin category when it makes us feel more active and heated – classically Yang characteristics. It does seem somewhat confusing, but let's look at what actually happens to our body when we drink coffee (caffeine). Essentially, this is where an extreme

Yang condition, (active mind, dynamic body) turns into an extreme Yin condition (depleted, drained mind and body).

We generally think of coffee as a "pick-me-up" and one that lasts a good couple of hours. Have you ever wondered why or how it does that?

It has to do with brain chemistry. Caffeine has a stimulating effect on the central nervous system. It stimulates our neuron firing, (brain-body messaging system); it increases blood sugar (brain-body fuel); and raises our metabolism (response time) to handle any "fight or flight" emergency situation that may arise. The challenge is that in our typical urban lifestyle, such life-threatening scenarios rarely happen. What does happen however, is we end up with a nice stash of "adrenaline-rich, blood sugar fuel" that would have ordinarily been used for such a fight or flight emergency. In the presence of this abundant blood sugar cache, we experience some wonderful benefits. These would include improved cognitive function, reaction time, mood and memory. It's the very reason why we desire an infusion of caffeine to perk us up in the morning and afternoon. The brain is not capable of storing blood sugar fuel, but instead depends on a "moment-to-moment infusion of blood sugar in order to function properly. But here's the clincher. After that high-octane fuel is expended, our body and brain are essentially left running on empty, and we feel drained and depleted. Sometimes we're so low in blood sugar fuel, our brain becomes foggy and our body is almost desperate for some replenishing fuel.

So, here's the mantra: it's all about balance. It's about paying attention to how we're feeling in our body, mind and emotions – and using the corrective measures of food or activity, to affect a specific or desired change.

When looking to balance a condition that's leaning toward the too-Yin side of the spectrum, the best remedy is utilizing some Yang-leaning or Yang-balancing guidelines. Here are some of those Yang-influencing recommendations that will help the body, mind and emotions feel more grounded, centered and stable.

> *Harmony is the ever-changing state of balancing the Yin and Yang energies within our body, lifestyle and environment.*

Healthy Yang-Influencing Guidelines:

- Serve foods warmed or heated.

- Sauté, bake, pressure-cook or slow simmer.

- Eat heartier protein.

- Include toasted, roasted or baked natural snacks (seeds, chips, crackers or popcorn).

- Eat sturdy, downward growing root vegetables.

- Use hearty, leafy green vegetables.

- Include tamari, Himalayan salt, miso or pickles.

- *Gomasio:* A toasted sesame and sea salt condiment used with veggies and grain. A small spoonful can help Yang-ize and support a more grounded sensation, when feeling too Yin.

- *Green Tea, Yerba Mate or Bancha/Kukicha twig tea:* Good for mental concentration, relieves fatigue, neutralizes acidity and alkalizes blood.

- *Ume extract tea:* (Ume plum *concentrate* – Eden brand. Not *salted* umeboshi plums). Very alkalizing, relieves upset stomach, hangover and liver congestion.

- *Ginger Root:* Freshly sliced or grated for tea, baking or stir fry. Stimulates sluggish intestines, promotes circulation and has heating qualities. Pickled ginger root is an excellent digestive aid.

- *Hard Cheeses:* When consuming dairy, a dry, hard, aged cheese, such as Parmesan, would be the least mucus producing and most Yang.

- *Coffee or Chai:* Any warm drink in general will make you feel better but coffee and Chai are especially known to have heating properties. Always best in moderation, or as espresso (smaller amount, less caffeine).

- *Garlic:* Acts as a thermo-genic, increasing both body temperature and metabolic rate.

- *Miso:* Aged, salty, soybean paste. Very grounding and very good for intestinal flora. (Hatcho miso is the most medicinally balancing.)

- *Black pepper:* Black pepper contains a compound called piperine, which has thermo-genic properties. Pepper is known to have anti-bacterial properties and is assistive with digestion and relieving gas.

- If you are low in iron, Nova Scotia Dulse tabs (Bernard Jensen Co.) are highly beneficial. While pregnant with my son, I took Dulse to boost my iron. Worked like a charm. I've taken it ever since. About 12-15 tablets a day.

IDENTIFYING YANG IMBALANCES WITHIN THE BODY

Similar to the noticeable symptoms associated with an imbalance of Yin energy – Yang symptoms of imbalance are as equally identifiable. The physical or bodily symptoms of being overly Yang include feeling heated, restless, "hyper" and tense. Emotionally we feel anxious, impatient, unstable and potentially explosive. This is where high blood pressure, tension headaches, irritability and explosive outbursts are experienced.

If you have any of the symptoms listed below, then you have patterns of heat and dryness to a greater or lesser degree – affecting both the body and the emotions.

Overly Yang Symptoms:
(Heat patterns or dry conditions)

- *Dry Conditions:* Dry rough skin, dry nasal passages, dry throat, dry eyes, dandruff and constipation
- Tendency to feel warm, heated in body. Drawn to cool-clothing attire
- Hyperactive, over-analyzing – always in motion, fast-talking
- Ruddier complexion. Rosy cheeks
- Prefers cold drinks, commonly thirsty
- Muscle tension. Sharp stitches, aches and pains in body
- High blood pressure. Nose bleeds
- Restless sleep, tosses and turns, disturbing dreams
- Prefers cooler climate
- Fever blisters, canker sores, bleeding gums, inflamed pimples

- Pressure headaches
- Night sweats, grinding of teeth
- Feeling irritable, impatient, defensive, stressed

Think of excess "Yang" patterning the way you would a pressure cooker that's slowly heating up. As the heat builds, so does the pressure – which needs to be relieved or an explosion will occur. This is precisely what happens in our own body. We operate at a high-stressed, "fiery" pace, while ingesting too many foods from the extreme Yang side of the spectrum (or not enough balancing Yin foods), and we ultimately create an over-heated, combustible, internal environment. This combustion has to be released in one way or another – and most typically manifests as emotional outbursts and behavior. Or worse. It can manifest as a complete physical breakdown or emotional burnout.

Let's look at how such a situation occurs. For experiment sake, let's say we choose to fast on a Yang diet consisting of eggs, hard cheese, meat, salty crackers, pretzels, chips and stimulating caffeinated energy-drinks – and maybe even add cigarettes to the mix. Let's say we did this for three weeks straight, all the while operating at a fairly aggravating, high-stressed pace. We're talking no veggies, fruits, salads, juices, sugary sweets or alcohol during this time. We might initially feel grounded and assertive with these foods, but with such a drying, warming kind of diet – combined with a heated, stressy, "jammin" pace – we would eventually find ourselves in a potentially combustible situation. As a balancing remedy, we would need to integrate some soothing, cooling and relaxing life force back into the body. We would need to lower the heat and release the pressure. Adding some cooling, moistening "Yin-leaning" foods and activity, along with a more integrated, gentler-paced, balanced lifestyle, would help achieve this.

Let's take a look at how a daily-life scenario could cause an overly Yang condition and pattern over time. Let's say for example, our work and familial obligations have become noticeably high-maintenance on every level. We have little enjoyment time for relationships, recreation, activities, vacation or even ourselves. On top of that, our finances are stretched to the max. It's no wonder we find ourselves feeling pressured, tightened-down and anxiety-filled.

In understanding the "Yang-patterned" pressure cooker analogy, we note a very similar response in the body as the adrenaline-stimulated cycle from caffeine. With such a stress-filled, overburdened lifestyle, our central nervous system is continually triggered in response to what the brain perceives as "emergency alerts" much as it does with caffeine. We're in a constant cycle of "priming the pump" to handle the taxing requirements of our life – and then afterwards, spiraling downward as the fuel runs out. If this exhausting and damaging cycle continues, not only will adrenal fatigue* set in, but related conditions such as chronic hypertension, heartburn, tension headaches, insomnia, muscular tightness and gastrointestinal issues are also apt to follow.

An interesting consideration to remember concerning the relationship between our body and emotions is, "as the body goes, so responds the emotions. As the emotions go, so registers the body."

* *The adrenals release the hormones that prepare the body to effectively handle emergencies.*

ADDRESSING IMBALANCED YANG SYMPTOMS

So, what do we do when we realize we've somehow crossed over into the land of extreme-Yang and are now responding to life and circumstances in a reactive manner? The simple answer is: Take a deep breath and *Slow. It. All. Down.*

Create the time and the space to *just be* in the moment of soft relaxation, peace and openness. Take slow deep breaths and remove yourself from the thoughts associated with the people, circumstances and responsibilities that got you jammed up in the first place. A good barometer of feeling spacious and balanced inside yourself is when you're able to easily take *full* deep breaths. When we're stressed, worried or anxious, we become tightened down in our chest (and belly) with a feeling of constriction. This "slow-it-all-down" practice will not only create a feeling of tranquility and stability in the body, but will also create a surplus of energetic Chi reserves.

When feeling "out of whack" and looking to balance a condition that we deem too-Yang, whether it's physical, mental or emotional, the one place we can make the most rapid and effective change is with our diet. We put our focus on implementing some Yin-leaning guidelines concerning food, preparation, environmental temperature and personal activity, thus supporting a revitalized perspective and demeanor.

Here are some of those Yin-influencing or "Yin-izing" guidelines that will encourage a more relaxed, refreshed and inspired body and mind:

Healthy Yin-Influencing Guidelines:

- Serve food cooler, raw, lightly steamed or cooked quickly in wok.

- *Raw mixed vegetable salad:* Spinach, cucumber, celery, sprouts, lettuce, beets and carrots.

- *Flowery, leafy, round vegetables:* Broccoli, cauliflower, cabbage, bok choy and chard.

- *Pod vegetables:* Snap peas, green beans and snow peas.

- *Summer squash:* Crookneck, zucchini and chayote.

- *Cooling whole grains:* Corn, barley, oatmeal, whole grain gluten-free pastas and breads.

- *Lighter proteins:* Tofu, tempeh, edamame, sprouted beans, quinoa and sushi/fish.

- Temperate raw fruits and juices such as apples, berries, strawberries, cherries, apricots and plums. When feeling balanced and strong, tropical fruits are just fine.

- *Cooling condiments:* Brown rice vinegar, apple cider vinegar, healthy mustard, mayo, salad dressings and ketchup.

- *Fermented dairy and dairy-like alternatives:* cow's milk, soy milk, coconut and almond milk-based yogurt and kefir, cultured butter and sour cream.

- Fresh vegetable juices.

- Bottled unsweetened fruit juices.

- Occasional beer, wine or spirits.

- Soft cheeses (moderately).

- *Raw or lightly roasted nuts and seeds:* Almonds, walnuts, filberts, pine nuts, pumpkin, sunflower and hemp seeds.

- Herbal cooling teas such as peppermint (assists with flatulence, digestion), white tea, green tea and chamomile (relaxes, aids sleep).

- Healthy, natural "sweets" (wholesome, clean ingredients, naturally sweetened).

- *Natural sweeteners:* Maple syrup, brown rice syrup, barley malt, Jerusalem artichoke syrup, yacon, coconut sugar/syrup, fruit-juice concentrate, Sucanat (organic whole sugar-cane), raw, dark agave and stevia.

COOKING AND PREPARING METHODS

Most Yang methods include dry heat, as in baking, and heat that involves increased pressure and additional cooking time. Yin methods of preparation include raw or refrigerated foods, quick stir-frying or steaming.

Here is the list from the most Yang method all the way down to the most Yin form of preparation:

- Baking
- Pressure cooking
- Casseroles or stews
- Roasting
- Deep-frying
- Sautéing
- Stir-frying
- Steaming
- Blanching
- Raw
- Chilled

Cooking in stainless steel, cast iron, glass, stoneware or good quality enamel is best. Aluminum can leach into your food, causing metal toxicity, which can cause stress to the kidneys. It can also transfer a metallic taste into your food. Also, when using any kind of coated pan such as Teflon, it's best not to use a high flame or high heat, as toxic gases are emitted at higher temperatures.

"The Bamboo that bends is stronger than the Oak that resists."

~ JAPANESE PROVERB

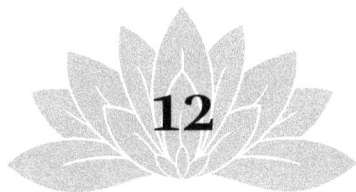

The Five Environmental Elements

After Yin-Yang Theory, the Five Element Theory was a natural evolution in Taoist philosophy. Prior to this system's inception, the natural phenomena of the world were most commonly observed and interpreted through the perspective of Yin and Yang.

By continually observing the cyclical patterns of nature, the ancient Taoists came to believe that five environmental or elemental forces governed the world. It was deduced that the elements of Water, Wood, Fire, Earth and Metal are the primary, energetic principles guiding our manifest world. The elements were understood to be transformative in nature. Each element has its own network of distinct attributes and interrelating patterns that influenced the cycles of birth, growth and decay; the shifting seasonal climatic conditions; human physiology, psychology and behavior; and the physical, medicinal and energetic properties of the very foods we eat.

The Five Element Theory focuses on the relationship between us and the cycles and elements of nature, and using these guiding principles to our greatest advantage. The Five Environmental Elements and their respective seasons provide a roadmap, indicating how to replenish the deficiencies and tone down the excesses, by effectively using a complementary food, flavor or method of preparation to nudge us back to center. When these elements are balanced and working effectively, our physical, mental and emotional health is abundant. This reciprocal relationship with nature influences our mental and emotional mood swings and impacts our body's function and performance. When in balance, this relationship can be to our greatest benefit, and when out of balance, to our unfortunate detriment. The practice of Feng Shui aspires to balance the five elements in a given environment, creating and supporting an atmosphere of harmony. Similarly, when the energy flow is disturbed or out of balance, disharmony occurs.

Cycle of Harmonious Transformation of the Elements:
(The cyclical movement and action of one Element affects and influences the next)

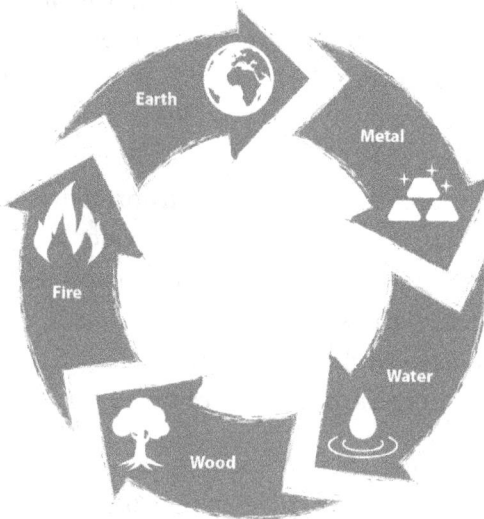

- **Wood** burns and fuels **Fire**
- **Fire** ash decomposes into **Earth**
- **Earth** gathers and houses **Metals**/minerals
- **Metals**/minerals enrich, infuse **Water**
- **Water** nourishes and grows **Wood**

Environmental Elements: Seasonal and Climatic Correspondences: (Climatic correspondences are external weather or environmental influences that effect or aggravate a physical or emotional condition.)

- **Wood** Element corresponds to the **Spring** season and a **Windy** environment.

  This is a time of birth, opportunity and new beginnings. During Spring, overly windy weather (or environment) can cause or aggravate imbalances in the body and emotions.

- **Fire** Element corresponds to the **Summer** season and a **Hot** environment.

  This is a time of activity, warmth, growth and relationship. During Summer, excessively hot weather (or environment) can cause or aggravate imbalances in the body and emotions.

- **Earth** Element corresponds to the **Late Summer** season and a **Damp** environment.

  This is a time of harvest, abundance, of reaping what we've sown. During Late Summer, excessively damp weather (or environment) can cause or aggravate imbalances in the body and emotions.

- **Metal** Element corresponds to the **Autumn** season and a **Dry** climate.

  This is a time of discarding, evaluating, slowing down for winter. During Autumn, excessively dry weather (or environment) can cause or aggravate imbalances in the body and emotions.

- **Water** Element corresponds to the **Winter** season and a **Cold** environment.

  This is a quieter time, of introspection, regrouping and rest. During Winter, excessively cold weather (or environment) can cause or aggravate imbalances in the body and emotions.

WATER	Winter	Cold
WOOD	Spring	Wind
FIRE	Summer	Heat
EARTH	Later Summer	Damp
METAL	Autumn	Dryness

WOOD ELEMENT AND SPRING

Wood (Tree) is the elemental energy associated with **Spring**, when new life, new growth, new opportunities and creative energy abound. It's a time of possibility for us to branch out, move toward our dreams, feeling grounded in our roots, yet easy and flexible in our attitude. Much like the supple branches of a great willow tree swaying in the wind, we aspire toward fluidity and agility in our body. That means making sure our muscles are well stretched, responsive, supple and relaxed at rest. We want our spine, joints and neck to feel aligned, limber and flexible.

This season has to do with spring-cleaning the body's main filter, the liver, to cleanse, detoxify, rejuvenate and boost functionality. Doing any type of exercise that causes a sweat is especially helpful. Also, drinking plenty of fluids; adding lemon or apple-cider vinegar to your water; adding moderate amounts of fermented or pickled foods, including dill pickles, yogurt, sauerkraut and kombucha; and including the herb Milk Thistle/Silymarin are all greatly assistive in purifying and nourishing the liver. It's best to sidestep the foods, beverages or habits that tend to tax the liver, such as high-fat or heavily fried foods, chemical or sugar-heavy processed foods, excessive alcohol and over-eating.

- **Season:** Spring. The first season of the year represents renewal, activity, growth and vitality. This is a time of opportunity, self-awareness and self-expression.

- **Activity:** Active exercises: hiking, biking, aerobics, anything that gets your heart rate up and helps you break a sweat.

- **Balancing and nourishing foods:** The ideal foods to eat in the spring are the sour-flavored foods that naturally grow during this season. This would include green-stalked veggies such as bok choy, chard, broccoli, scallions, spinach, asparagus, celery and sprouts. Fruits would include Granny-Smith apples, plums, pineapple and citrus fruits, especially lemons, oranges and grapefruit. Any kind of sour or fermented foods such as yogurt, kefir, sourdough bread, Kombucha tea and all kinds of pickled foods including Kim chi, sauerkraut and olives.

It's a time to reduce or eliminate high-fat and rich foods and also reduce portion size. Smaller meals more often work well during this season. Spring is a good time to introduce a cleansing, cooling raw foods diet.

- **Taste or flavor**: Sour. Sour foods, such as vinegars, pickles, sauerkraut, lemon and ume plum extract, move energy inwards and tone the body's tissues. The sour flavor is most active in the liver where it counteracts the effects of excessively rich, heavy and greasy food, acting as a solvent in breaking down fats and proteins. The sour flavor tends to have a refreshing and enlivening effect on our taste buds.

- **Cooking/storing method**: Steaming, blanching, searing, grilling, campfire cooking, smoking, fermenting or pickling. As we adjust our somewhat heavier, winter-weather, cooking style to the lighter, spring-weather style, we assist in the release of proteins and fats, previously stored in the liver during the colder, winter months.

- **Climatic correspondence**: Wind (if you are imbalanced, being out in the windy weather can be aggravating physically or emotionally).

- **Balanced positive emotions**: With a strong liver and gall bladder, we possess patience, confidence, initiative, good-judgment and forgiveness.

- **Imbalanced negative emotions**: Anger, resentment, impatience, frustration, arrogance and impulsiveness.

- **Bodily organ**: Liver and gall bladder. The liver plays an important part in our body's digestive and filtration system. Everything we ingest, including medicines, drugs, chemical additives, acetaminophen or alcohol, is filtered through the liver. Of equal importance, the liver regulates our hormones, enzymes and blood sugar levels; it manufactures bile for the digestion of fats; it metabolizes nutrients into stored blood sugar fuel; and it also produces proteins needed for blood clotting. The gall bladder stores the bile produced by the liver, which, when imbalanced, can become crystallized, resulting in the formation of gallstones.

- **Common physical imbalance**: Liver stagnation. Stagnation occurs when a diet is consistently filled with foods that are considered rich and greasy – mammal meats, fats, intoxicants, eggs, cheese and refined foods – causing the liver to become sluggish and swollen. As the taxed, expanded liver continually struggles to do its job, heat is generated, causing not only negative emotional imbalances, but also physical ones such as migraines, dizziness, dry/inflamed eyes, acne/boils, inflexible muscles/ligaments/tendons and overall bodily dryness.

FIRE ELEMENT AND SUMMER

As the spring turns into **Summer**, we arrive at the most energetic phase of the cycle, the **Fire** element. This is a time of flourishing dynamism, full of warmth and activity. We have the stimulating heat from the summer sun; our bodies feel vitally energized; we're more physically active, more socially engaged; and we feel more connected to our family, friends and partners.

The summer season is associated with the fire of passion, love, generosity, joy, compassion and openness. Understandably, this seasonal energy relates to the heart and cardiovascular system, which is also associated with our emotional temperament.

The heart is the organ most responsible for sustaining life, by pumping and circulating nutrient-rich blood throughout our body. When we combine poor dietary practices such as excessive fat, sugar and processed foods, along with a sedentary lifestyle, it causes our blood to become viscous and sludgy, our organs to become swollen and labored, and our arterial walls to become lined (and narrowed) with fatty-deposits and plaque build-up. Once the pipes get clogged, we are at risk for arterial disease, high blood pressure, high cholesterol, heart attacks, shortness of breath, panic attacks and nervous disorders.

- **Season:** Summer. A time of the year representing growth, expansion, buoyancy, outward activity and creativity. This is the time of the year when we are out socializing, entertaining and doing activities with friends and family.

- **Activity:** This is a time best suited for anything involving aerobic or cardio activity.

- **Balancing and cooling/nourishing foods:** The ideal foods to eat in the summer are foods that are red in color, dried, hot and spicy. Think Mexican food: tomatoes, salsa, corn, bell peppers, scallions, hot chili peppers, black pepper, cayenne pepper. Any of the bitter-flavored lettuces are good, especially arugula, endive, romaine, watercress and bitter sprouts.

- Other Fire/Summer energy foods are asparagus, brussels sprouts, quinoa, rhubarb, apricots, cherry, persimmon, plums and kumquats. These foods can help reduce heat and assist with circulation.

  If per chance you're experiencing too much heat in your system, then cooling foods such as cucumber, yogurt, citrus, sprouts, watermelon, pears and apples can be assistive. Beer and wine, coffee, tea and carbonated beverages have all been found to help disperse excess heat in our bodies. Amounts are left up to your intuitive discretion. Moderation is key.

- **Taste or flavor:** Bitter. Bitter foods have a drying action, and energetically, move downward. The bitter flavor is identified with the heart, where it clears and cleanses arteries of mucous, cholesterol and fatty deposits. It has been known to assist in lowering blood pressure.

- **Cooking/storing method:** Stir-frying, flash or deep-frying, sautéing, toasting, pan roasting and dehydrating. The cooking styles become lighter and faster. Appetizers, stir-fries and snacks are prevalent at this time of the year, as we find ourselves socializing, entertaining and being more physically active.

- **Climatic correspondence:** Heat (if you are imbalanced, being out in the hot sun can exacerbate a physical or emotional condition).

- **Balanced positive emotions:** With a strong heart and small intestine we feel calm and easy, joyous, enthusiastic, openhearted and passionate.

- **Imbalanced negative emotions:** Agitated, stressed, competitive, pressured, confused and uncomfortably vulnerable.

- **Bodily organ:** Heart and small intestine. Heart-mind. In the Chinese medical definition, the heart not only regulates and propels blood circulation, but also houses the mind/spirit and affects the quality of consciousness, memory and sleep.

- **Common physical imbalance:** Thickened and sluggish blood, fluid and Chi flow, throughout the cardiovascular system and heart. Balancing and healing remedy: A simple "clean" diet with lunch as your main meal. Eating less, with occasional fasting, will contribute greatly toward calming and focusing the mind, as will avoiding or eliminating late-night eating, large evening meals, excessive coffee, refined sugar, alcohol and mucous-forming, rich foods. Whole grains – brown rice and oats, chewed well – contribute greatly toward calming the mind.

EARTH ELEMENT AND LATE SUMMER

Toward the end of summer comes the shorter season of **Late Summer** (Indian Summer) – a time of transition and balance – when the **Fire** energy has now burned down and mellowed, and returns to Earth energy. This is the calming, steady, balance point of the elemental and seasonal cycle between the more Yang cycle of Spring and Summer and the more Yin cycle of Fall and Winter. Respectively, this is a time of feeling grounded, centered and easy within ourselves – where we experience a sense of well-being and balance.

The organs associated with Earth energy are the stomach, spleen and pancreas – centered in the body managing the delicate balance between digestion, nourishment and blood sugar levels. When this delicate equilibrium becomes compromised, the digestive process, assimilation and distribution of nutrients are hampered, thereby affecting our vitality.

- **Season:** Late Summer. A pleasant, tranquil and flourishing time of the year. Promotes unity, harmony, comfort, centeredness, security and a balanced "middle-way" path.

- **Activity:** Mellow movement. Walking, hiking in nature, camping.

- **Balancing and nourishing foods:** The ideal foods to eat during the Indian or late summer months are the sweet flavored foods that are yellow and orange in color. Starchy root vegetables such as carrots, sweet potato, yam, potato, okra, beets, winter and summer squashes, cucumber, cabbage and cooked sweet onion are in this category. Sweet, soft fruits and nuts include cantaloupe, watermelon, sweet apples, grapes, peaches, sweet cherries, papayas, mangos, dates, banana, coconut and almonds. The best grains during this time would be barley, corn, oats and millet.

  If you are desirous of sweets, the best choices would be maple syrup, brown rice syrup, raw agave syrup or barley malt syrup. Earth foods assist with digestion, assimilation and neutralizing toxins. If you're feeling out of whack with digestion, if your Chi feels sluggish or if you're tired all the time, it's best to eat foods that have *thermogenic* or warming qualities, such as whole grains, plant-based protein, vegetables and cooked or baked seasonal fruits. Pungent spices such as: ginger, onion, garlic, leek, fennel, cinnamon, nutmeg and black pepper are assistive.

- **Taste/flavor:** Sweet. Sweet foods moisten, harmonize and nourish. Mildly sweet vegetables: corn, carrots, parsnip, cabbage, peas, sweet potatoes, winter squash and string beans. Green, yellow or golden colored foods. Seasonal fruits: cantaloupe, apricots and cherries. Legumes: garbanzos and yellow lentils.

- **Cooking/storing method:** Poaching, baking, roasting, stewing and "crock-pot" style cooking. The making of jams, jellies, candies and sweet desserts.

- **Climatic correspondence:** Dampness (if you are imbalanced, being out in the damp weather can exacerbate a physical or emotional condition).

- **Balanced positive emotions:** With a strong spleen, pancreas and stomach, our nature tends to be more nurturing, compassionate, stable, contented, sympathetic and considerate.

- **Imbalanced negative emotions:** Self-absorption, worry, self-doubt, neediness, indecisiveness and nervousness.

- **Bodily organ:** Stomach, spleen and pancreas. These organs are responsible for effective digestion of food, assimilation and distribution of nutrients. The resulting energetic essence from these organs functioning properly is strong immunity, vitality, orderliness, warmth, nurturing of self and others and a creative and centered mind.

- **Common physical imbalance:** Deficient Chi energy. Chronically tired, general weakness, anemia, ulcers, body lethargy, sluggishness, abdominal lumps, poor digestion, feeling mentally and physically "stuck" and tending toward a messy or cluttered environment. Damp condition in and of the body. Tendency toward moist accumulation or condition in body, such as edema, cysts, tumors, bloated abdomen and being overweight without excessively eating. Tendency toward the overgrowth of bacteria, yeast, viruses and parasites.

METAL ELEMENT AND AUTUMN

As late summer moves into the **Autumn** season, the days become shorter and the energy begins to contract and draw inward, indicating a completion cycle. It's the perfect time for crops to be harvested and stored, and for us to begin winding down in preparation for winter. The prior Earth energy, now transforms into **Metal** energy. Think of the minerals and precious metals that come from the earth. It's a time of purification, elimination and refinement; a time of internal reflection, contemplation and reorganization; of letting go of old habitual patterns that no longer serve us. The purifying organs associated with Metal energy are the lungs and large intestines. The lungs purify and utilize air, and the intestines rid our body of waste. You'll recognize you're getting off-balance if you begin feeling susceptible to respiratory problems. These would include difficulty with breathing, coughs, colds, flu, asthma, pneumonia and excess phlegm. You may also notice abnormalities in your bowels, such as constipation or diarrhea. Bowel cleansings, vigorous pranayamic breath work and dry saunas can be very assistive at this time.

- **Season:** Autumn. A time of fullness, preparation and organization, of gathering and drawing into oneself. In nature, this is a time of contraction. The life force stops flowing from the roots to the outer branches. Leaves fall and fruit dries up. As the seeded fruit or pods fall to the ground, a new cycle will begin in the fertile springtime.

- **Activity:** In this season of cleansing and refining, it's a good time to get rid of anything that is not necessary, useful or contributing to your life. Mentally and spiritually focused practices, as well as refined physical activity, can be highly assistive in reassessing, culling and streamlining your life.

- **Balanced and nourishing foods:** The ideal foods for the Fall season are savory, hearty vegetables, grains, beans and some meat, if desired. Veggies such as carrots, cauliflower, parsnips, potatoes, pumpkin, onion, garlic, mustard greens, radish, daikon, turnip and winter squashes are good, as are whole grains such as short-grain brown rice, autumn corn and millet. All white beans are recommended, such as Great Northern, Navy and soybeans, including tofu and tempeh. Savory mushrooms, such as shitake and porcini help with eliminating mucus and phlegm. Herbs and spices, such as cayenne, cinnamon, cilantro, cloves, curry, fennel, ginger, horseradish, spinach, tarragon, mustard, nutmeg, parsley, pepper, rosemary, scallions, thyme, wasabi and watercress, are all considered eliminative and cleansing. Recommended seasonal fruits are pears, apples, grapes, mangoes and bananas.

Metal-foods benefit us when we're feeling cold, sluggish, damp and lethargic. They tend to have a dispersing effect on bodily stagnation, a drying effect on dampness, and also activate the circulation of Chi flow. They will assist with any anomalies of the lungs, respiration and bowel function.

- **Taste/flavor:** Pungent. Pungent foods move energy from the center to the surface, stimulate circulation, disperse stagnation and tend to be drying. These would include: garlic, ginger, radishes and mustard.

- **Cooking method:** Baking and pressure-cooking. Mincing, dicing and the inclusion of garnishes and condiments.

- **Climatic correspondence:** Dryness (if you are imbalanced, being in a dry climate can be aggravating physically or emotionally).

- **Balanced positive emotions:** With strong healthy lungs and large intestines, we feel integrated, directed, orderly, self-reflective, focused, courageous and clear.

- **Imbalanced negative emotions:** Grief, depression, regret, defeat and rigidity.

- **Bodily organ:** Lungs and large intestines. Utilizing the vital Chi from the air we breathe and combining it with the energetic-nutrients extracted from the food we eat, the lungs produce, distribute and maintain a moist, protective coating on all mucous membranes, and promote soft, lustrous, well-nourished skin and hair. A person with healthy lungs has a strong immunity from viruses, bacteria, colds, flu and invading pathogens.

- **Common physical imbalance:** The most typical challenge when the lungs are imbalanced is poor respiration. In the colon, it manifests as congestion and constipation. This is generally caused by a more sedentary lifestyle, accompanied by a diet filled with congesting foods, such as dairy, meat, processed foods and cigarettes. Unresolved grief and sadness are the common emotional challenges linked to these organs.

WATER ELEMENT AND WINTER

Water is the elemental energy associated with **Winter**, when dormancy, gestation and potential prevail. The winter is a time when everything slows down. It's a quieter time of rest, relaxation, reading, writing and inward reflection, when all forms of life energetically begin gathering, condensing, conserving and storing for the stark and barren months ahead. In our body, the water element is understandably related to all fluids: blood circulation, the lymph system, the bladder, perspiration, tears, and most importantly, the kidneys. As was discussed earlier, the kidneys are essentially our energy banks, where Chi reserves are generated, stored and utilized. It's especially important in the winter to keep our kidneys healthy, hydrated and warmly heated. Warming foods like hot, savory soups, stews, slow-burning whole grains, Yang-leaning root vegetables, nutrient-rich greens, roasted nuts and seeds, black, kidney or adzuki beans, and warming drinks such as grated ginger, cinnamon and chai-spice teas are the ideal foods for this season.

- **Season:** Winter. This is a time of introspection, receptiveness, re-evaluation, self-nurturing, and a time to foster your dreams, visions and opportunities.

- **Activity:** Important to keep your Yang energy fired up. It's critical to feel securely heated in your center or core. Engage in more "fluid/flowing" easy activity, such as hot baths, walks, dance movement, yoga, Tai Chi or Qigong. Skiing can also be a good choice. Anything that gets you feeling warm from the inside out, helps with circulation and keeping your Chi balanced – is a good thing.

- **Balancing and warming/nourishing foods:** Salty foods and dark-colored foods are included in this category. Seasonings such as miso, tamari and sea salt; sea foods such as seaweeds, fresh and salted fish, caviar and shellfish; black beans, kidney beans and adzuki beans, wild rice, short-grain brown rice and buckwheat, eggs, walnuts, black sesame seeds and fruits and veggies such as blueberries, blackberries, eggplant and kale will all assist in grounding and holding energy and heat in our bodies. Winter is the perfect time to introduce root vegetable's slow burning and centering energy into our diet. These foods have a softening and calming effect on us emotionally and assist in thickening the blood to keep the body core warmed.

- **Taste/flavor:** Salty. Salty foods draw energy downward, moistening, detoxifying and promoting a grounded feeling in the body.

- **Cooking/storing method:** Boiling, simmering, steaming, poaching, curing and freezing.

- **Climatic correspondence:** Coldness (if you are imbalanced, being out in the cold weather can be aggravating physically or emotionally).

- **Balanced positive emotions:** Inspiration, flexibility, courage, wisdom, willpower, trust and endurance are indicative of having a strong, healthy and balanced kidney and bladder.

- **Imbalanced negative emotions:** Fear, doubt, disinterest, resignation and despondency are the emotions associated with an imbalanced kidney or bladder.

- **Bodily organ:** Kidneys and bladder.

- **Common physical imbalance:** Dark circles under eyes or puffiness, low back pain, adrenal exhaustion and chronic urinary-tract problems.

How Your Emotions Affect Your Health
(Bolded emotion is dominant. Non-bolded is secondary emotion)

- **Anger.** Resentment: Weakens/Aggravates the **Liver** and **Gall Bladder.**

- **Grief.** Depression: Weakens/Aggravates the **Lungs** and **Large Intestines.**

- **Worry.** Self-doubt: Weakens/Aggravates the **Stomach**, **Spleen** and **Pancreas.**

- **Stress.** Agitation: Weakens/Aggravates the **Heart** and **Mind.**

- **Fear.** Despondency: Weakens/Aggravates the **Kidneys** and **Bladder.**

Part Four
Application and Refinement

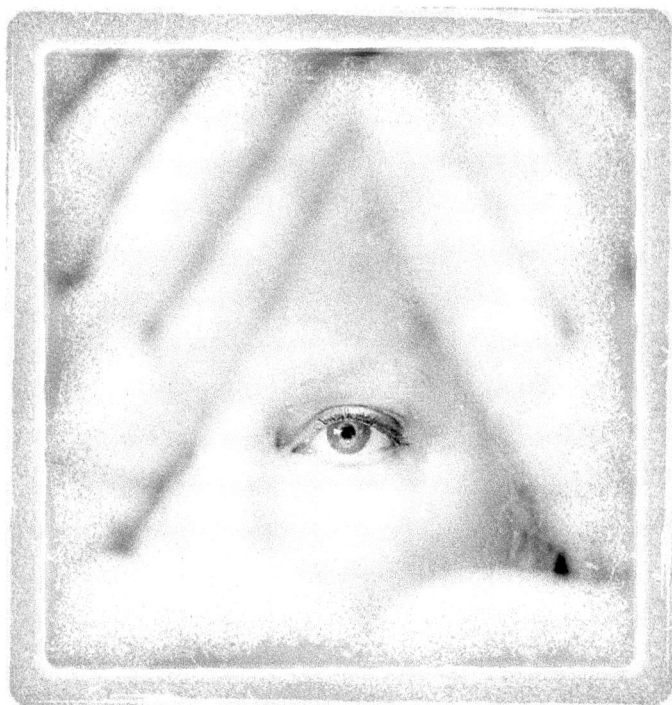

"Mindfulness: The practice of paying attention...on purpose...in the present moment...nonjudgmentally."

~ JON KABAT-ZINN

13

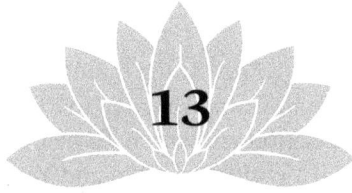

Self-Inquiry and Assessment

"If we do not change our direction, we are likely to
end up where we are headed."
– ANCIENT CHINESE PROVERB

Similar to the cycles within nature, we live according to the
cycles of our human existence – those within our body, our
relationships, our ideas and our personal evolution. We
have a beginning cycle of discovery and growth. We have a
dynamic cycle of journeying through life's experiences. And,
we have a more seasoned cycle of maturation, enjoying the
fruits of our labor and living a more preferential life.

We are an ever-unfolding "work in progress," experiencing
and awakening unto life. And while we sincerely endeavor
to be our most healthfully balanced self, there are always
going to be those times, as within nature, when erratic and
unpredictable occurrences happen. When they do, it's very
empowering to know how to respond and effectively bring
ourselves back into balance.

"Thus, *Knowing How* is the maintenance of Life.
To observe the Seasons, To adapt to Heat and Cold,
To Harmonize elation and anger, To be Calm in activity,
as in rest. To regulate the Yin and Yang, And,
to Balance the hard and soft."
– THE YELLOW EMPEROR'S CLASSIC OF MEDICINE,
THE NEI JING SU WEN.[9]

The Nei Jing is one of the most important classic texts of Taoism. To the ancient Taoists, it gave practical advice on how to maintain balance by working with the rhythmic and esoteric laws of nature. It spoke to how our environment, lifestyle, diet and temperament all have an effect on our health: and how the external influences around us, such as the changing seasons, climate and geography, all have a corresponding influence on our internal emotions and behavior.

To be able to apply such wisdom, we must first understand and experience what it feels like to be *in* balance, so we can easily recognize when our body, emotions and lives become out of balance. Sometimes these imbalances come to our awareness on the emotional or mental level, when we feel somewhat "off" and out of sorts. We're not as confident, clear thinking or in the flow as we're used to feeling. Other times it hits us on the physical level, where the usual efficiency, ease and groundedness in our body starts to feel sluggish, impeded or resistant in some way.

I have found that the quickest and most effective way to address any imbalance is on the physical level. This is where we have the most control and can effect the greatest change simply by altering our diet and lifestyle. It's much more challenging and considerably less effective to try and resolve the emotional issues and imbalances when the physical body is out of whack.

> *The quickest and most effective way to address an imbalance is by altering our diet. This is where we have the most control and can effect the greatest change.*

So, how do we develop this instinctive awareness? One of the best ways to awaken or engage our instincts is through the practice of self-inquiry. We do this as if we are attempting to contact an old friend whom we've not talked to in a while. We want to open up the lines of communication to see what's going on and get a pulse. For us personally, the intention is to check in – see how we are doing and what we are feeling – in our physical, emotional and mental being. Most of the time, this interchange is already going on as we register various assessments and input. We're just not always mindful of it. There is unparalleled wisdom residing within us, just waiting to be tapped. The way to tap into this cache of wisdom and use it to our utmost advantage is by fostering the symbiotic relationship between our inner knowing and our conscious mind. This is a very doable objective.

> "Excellence is never an accident. It is always the result of high intention, sincere effort and intelligent execution; it represents the wise choice of many alternatives – choice, not chance, determines your destiny."
> – ARISTOTLE

When first beginning the practice of self-inquiry, you will find yourself automatically doing quick assessments throughout the day, especially before meals. The easiest time to start is in the morning before getting out of bed. It's a softer, slower time, well suited for contemplation and meditation – especially before we "kick it in" and start our day.

It goes something like this: Upon waking, softly, slowly and deeply – *inhale.* Luxuriate. Smile. Smiling has an alchemical effect on our psyche. It really does. Take a moment to acknowledge all of the wonderful blessings in your life, because for each of us, there is much to be thankful for. Rest in the appreciation and knowledge that *you are good.*

A shift in perception will not only alter your attitude, but will completely change your bodily response.

Then a simple self-inquiry: How am I feeling today? Do I feel easy with myself, or am I unsettled? What's going on in my body? Do I feel good and strong today or do I have the "slows?" Do I feel clear-headed or foggy brained? You get the picture. It's about initiating an inner dialogue to uncover and identify your varying moods, feelings, observations and reactions. These are all very good indicators of how you're handling the circumstances around you. This process of self-inquiry is a way of awakening and engaging your most instinctive self – no more responding or functioning on automatic pilot.

Self-Inquiry is a good barometer of how you're managing the circumstances around you, both physically and emotionally. It's an exercise to awaken and engage your most instinctive self.

You will also want to give some thought to any required outlay of energy, be it physically or mentally. Will you be doing something that requires physical exertion and stamina? How about something that requires that you bring your clearest and sharpest mind to the table? Or, is it a relatively mellow day with plenty of options and space?

> *The secret to effecting change is to focus on what you want, rather than what you don't want.*

What self-inquiry does is cultivate a connection between our habit-oriented (auto-pilot) mind and our instinctual self. We're able to tap in, do a quick assessment, and then effectively use our food to alter or support our present standing. Knowing intuitively what foods to eat, how they should be prepared and when they best serve our particular needs, is an evolving practice that does become easier with time.

OPENING UP A DIALOGUE BETWEEN THE MIND AND BODY

> *The more you encourage and engage your intuition, the stronger, clearer and more accurate it becomes.*

1. Assessments of Mood and Body Upon Waking

Today, I am feeling in my body or emotions:

A. Balanced

B. Too Yin

C. Too Yang

If you're feeling good and balanced within yourself, you can eat just about anything. If you're feeling too Yin, lean toward grounding and strengthening Yang foods. If you are feeling more Yang, lighten up your diet with some fresh, moistening and cooling Yin foods.

A. **Balanced:** Feeling easy, light-hearted, relaxed, happy, intuitive, loving, optimistic, vital, connected, appreciative, creative, sensitive, open, curious, motivated, energized, focused, centered, productive and positive. Feeling good and supported, feeling tuned-in and at-one-with my environment, life and loved ones.

   When we are balanced, we can eat just about anything we want and participate in just about any activity we choose.

B. **Too Yin:** Feeling "flat," fatigued and passive: Mind and body feel "removed," tired, vulnerable, separate, depressed, low energy, spacey, chilled, flu-like, insecure, melancholy, pessimistic, disappointed, procrastinating and weepy. Not really up for much of anything. Sluggish, not motored. *Need to fire up.*

   A more Yang, heated, grounding kind of meal would be best. Get outside, in nature, and do some kind of cardio activity – anything that gets your heart rate up.

C. **Too Yang:** Feeling tight, anxious and reactive: mind and body feel tightly wound, restless, achy, tense, heated up, edgy, irritated, defensive, frustrated, trapped, angry and aggressive. Great potential for burnout or meltdown. *Time to chill out, relax and cool down.*

A more Yin, raw, cooling kind of meal would be most balancing, in addition to mellow activity, such as yoga, swimming, walking and anything involving nature.

2. Assessment of Energetic Requirement or Outlay

Today, my physical or mental energy/output will be:

A. Balanced

B. More Yin

C. More Yang

A. **Balanced:** Everything is easily handled or manageable as far as energy output. You can easily accommodate today's energy requirement, whatever it is. You feel energetically and emotionally upbeat, physically strong, mentally capable and up for handling anything that presents itself.

B. **More Yin:** Today's requirement is relatively low-key and has a spacious, relaxed flow to it. Comfortable, casual and stress-free. Lot's of options. Think: laidback, easy-going weekend or vacation.

C. **More Yang:** Today is going to require a major amount of focused and directed energy. It is a dynamically active or strenuous day – be it physically or mentally.

3. Assessment of Weather

Different types of weather affect the way we feel, dress, eat, move, behave and perform. Check on the weather and see how it matches up with how you're feeling physically, mentally and emotionally. Eat accordingly.

A. **Balanced:** What we refer to as perfect weather. A day that makes you want to be outside. The temperature is great and the air is clean. You are buoyantly optimistic and your mood and physical vitality mirrors the weather outside. Eat whatever type of foods you're drawn to.

B. **More Yin:** Cooler, colder temperatures. Damp, wet, stormy or snowy. These are the kind of days you want to "cozy-down" by a warm fire, soak in a hot bath or relax with a good book. A more Yang leaning diet is typically desired.

C. **More Yang:** Sunny, hot, humid or dry. Think 100-degree weather. OK to do just about anything; however, hydration and Chi preservation are very important. More hydrating, raw and cooling fruits, veggies and juices are usually in order.

"What purifies you
is the right road."
~ RUMI

14

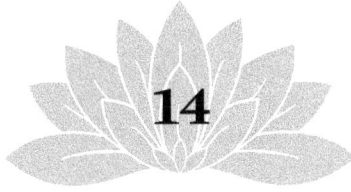

Daily Implementation

Optimal health is the harmonious alignment of body, mind, emotions and behavior – rather than simply the absence of disease.

- *Upon first awakening each morning, drink 8-10 oz. of water* with some freshly squeezed lemon or organic lemon juice concentrate.

- *Upon awakening: smile, inhale deeply, be appreciative, do a quick, soft assessment of how you're feeling on all levels.* Choose a complementary balancing and supporting meal. If you've got Yin watery symptoms, like a runny nose, allergies, phlegm, bloating or feeling foggy-headed and lethargic, it's best to go for more Yang heat-producing foods that will help dry up the excess fluid. If you've got Yang tightening, pressured or heated symptoms like a headache, high blood pressure or are feeling stressed and reactionary, it's best to eat, drink or snack on something that moistens and cools down the dry, Yang heat.

> *Warm lemon water serves as the perfect first morning-beverage. It alkalizes the digestive system, flushes out body toxins, purifies the blood, supports the immune system and makes it much easier for the body to eliminate any waste products.*

- *Whenever possible, do your best to consume only **organic** fruits, veggies, grains, beans, nuts, seeds, eggs, poultry and meat.* Many of the larger grocery store chains now carry organic and locally grown "clean" foods, as do local natural food stores and farmers' markets. Animal meats and by-products are best consumed when they are from animals that are organically raised, pasture-fed and free-range, and without any added antibiotics or hormones.

Organic products are:

- Made without irradiated products or ingredients.

- Made without artificial preservatives, coloring, flavoring or chemical additives.

- Made without monosodium glutamate (MSG), aspartame, sodium nitrates or nitrites.

- Made without genetically modified organisms (GMO).

> "Every major food company now has an organic division. There is more capital going into organic agriculture than ever before."
> – MICHAEL POLLAN

- *Include healthy fats in your diet, especially in their natural form – as they appear in nature.* Raw nuts, seeds, avocados, naturally processed olives, pasture-fed, whole-milk dairy products and fish sources are all rich in Omega-3 essential fatty acids.

Including healthy fats in your diet boosts metabolism,
helps absorb nutrients, encourages fat-burning,
curbs cravings, supports immunity and
provides stabilized energy.

- *When including dairy products in your diet, it is best to go for the easy-to-digest, probiotic rich and fermented varieties, such as yogurt, kefir, sour cream and cultured butter.* The fermentation or culturing process produces beneficial probiotics and enzymes that make the dairy easier to digest. As far as cheeses go, the drier, saltier and aged types are considered more Yang, more grounding and less mucus forming.

Fermented foods are rich in digestive enzymes
and beneficial bacteria to help improve digestive
health, fortify the immune system and assist with
digestion, absorption and utilization of nutrients from
the foods we eat.

- *Include naturally fermented foods in your diet – daily.* Adding a small amount of these foods to your diet will help produce beneficial enzymes and probiotic bacteria that will assist with immunity, digestion, body/organ detoxification and overall health and well-being. Examples include Kombucha tea, yogurt, kefir, pickles, sauerkraut, kim-chi, tempeh and miso.

Kombucha tea has beneficial yeasts that have been shown to improve digestion, nutrient assimilation, immunity, and to help fight candida overgrowth.

- *When drinking bottled fruit juices, choose beverages whose labels indicate 100 percent juice, as opposed to a fruit "drink."* The word "drink" usually implies added fructose, sugar, artificial flavorings or ingredients. Keep in mind that even 100 percent juice, whether bottled or freshly pressed, is still a very concentrated form of natural sugar. We would be hard pressed to eat 5-10 carrots or 3-4 apples in one sitting and that's the sugar equivalent in the pressed juice. It is best to consume no more than 8-10 ounces at one sitting.

- *Pure, young coconut water, harvested from green coconuts, is a refreshing and hydrating alternative.* I find the coconuts from Thailand to contain the best tasting water, and even those have varying levels of sweetness. Check the label for 100 percent pure coconut water, without any added ingredients or sugar. Make sure the coconut water is not made from a reconstituted concentrate. What is the point in eliminating the organic coconut water's nutrients and beneficial enzymes, and instead adding denatured city water?

Young coconut water is a sweet tasting, exceptionally
hydrating fluid taken from young-green coconuts.
A healthy balance of electrolytes, minerals, enzymes
and B vitamins makes it well suited to regulate,
replenish and rehydrate the body's fluid levels during
hot temperatures, exercise, intestinal illness
and electrolyte imbalance.

- *Simple carbohydrates are best reduced and preferably eliminated from your daily diet.* These would include the more processed and refined white flours, white sugars, white rice, white pastas and white peeled potatoes – yep, all the "white" stuff. Complex carbohydrates are the preferred choice with items such as whole grains, vegetables, fruits, legumes (best sprouted) and raw, soaked or lightly toasted seeds and nuts.

Complex carbs are foods whose nutrients, enzymes
and sugars are broken down slowly and efficiently
and used by the body as nourishment and fuel. Simple
carbs are the "white" refined, non-nutritive foods that
infuse the body with empty calories that
eventually turn to fat.

- *Move your body, in some way, every day, even for short periods.* Do something that gets your heart rate up and something that causes you to sweat. It can be any level of housework, yard work, isometrics, dancing, cardio, sprinting or full-on marathoning. Any outdoor activity, whether hiking in nature, walking, biking, swimming, jogging or gardening, can make a huge difference in how you look and feel in your body. Being outdoors in the fresh air and sun invigorates and boosts your natural defenses.

Every single system in the body is refreshed and revitalized by daily exercise – from the respiratory, circulatory, digestive, nervous, endocrine and immune system, to the muscular, skeletal and integumentary (hair, skin, nails) system.

- *Hot Epsom salt baths, saunas and steams are a wonderfully balancing addition to our daily routine, especially when the immune system needs boosting or when the body's core feels chilled.* They are an extremely effective and relaxing therapy for the body and mind. Epsom salts (magnesium sulfate) flush the lactic acid out of overworked or sore muscles and actually help detoxify the body. Adding apple cider vinegar to baths is also very cleansing and alkalizing. The vinegar smell evaporates quickly.

An Epsom salt bath not only helps replenish magnesium levels, it helps eliminate toxins, reduce inflammation, relieve muscular cramps, relax the nervous system, alleviate stress, soften skin and improve blood circulation in the body.

- *Accentuate the things you like doing that bring passion and joy into your life – that "light you up" and make you smile.* Hang out with the people who stimulate and fuel your curiosity; who inspire you and make you want to be better and do well. Laugh out loud. A lot. Be thankful. The thoughts you entertain and the company you keep effect you on every level.

*Dietary portions have increased by at least four times
since the 1950s. The "average" adult today is 26+
pounds heavier than 60 years ago.*

- *Consider the practice of caloric-consciousness, as best epitomized by the long-living healthy cultures in Chapter 7.* It's not about restricting our food intake, but being conscious of when we're comfortably full. Think about the 80 percent rule. It's actually an easy practice to implement. You begin by simply taking smaller portions. You can always go back for more. Next, slowly savor your food. Lastly, you'll want to familiarize yourself with what it means to be "reasonably and comfortably" full.

*Adequate sleep strengthens immunity, reduces stress,
bolsters memory, promotes healing, boosts creativity
and enhances physical performance.*

- *Get an adequate, restful amount of sleep.* It's been shown that much of our rejuvenating and regenerative healing goes on during sleep.

- *Shoot for a solid 7-9 hours of sleep, if at all possible.* It's been said that the hours before 12 midnight count as double. Going to bed at 10 gives you the equivalent of four hours of sleep before the midnight hour.

"Sleep is the best meditation."
– DALAI LAMA

"*Knowing yourself is the beginning of all Wisdom.*"

~ ARISTOTLE

15

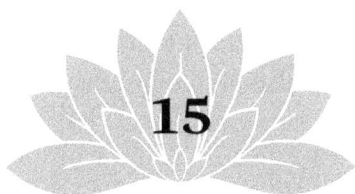

Restorative Practices

"The best time to plant a tree was 20 years ago.
The next best time is now."
– CHINESE PROVERB

Here are some very simple and effective relaxation practices that will initiate a calmer, healthier and more integrated mental and physical state. We all have a natural, innate relaxation response within the body. The goal is to trigger that response with simple relaxation exercises.

SIMPLE GRATITUDE MEDITATION: A FEW MINUTES, TWICE A DAY

Upon waking... slowly, softly and deeply inhale and exhale. Smile – yes, smile. Smiling has an absolutely positive effect on the body's chemistry. You can actually feel it. Stretch. Luxuriate. Give thanks for your life and the day yet to unfold. Allow yourself to have a few moments of easy, relaxed curiosity and contemplation, for what might, what could, happen today. Set your positive tone right now. What do I feel, think and envision when imagining a "good day?" This is a simple proactive form of meditation that will set the tone for the rest of your day. It's also incredibly easy to do.

> *Smiling has an opening, encouraging and positive effect on our physiology and psychology. It's a highly beneficial practice. The more you do it, the better you'll feel.*

Engage in the same appreciation contemplation before nodding off to sleep. Take a deep inhalation and a slow exhalation. Softly smile with an attitude of gratitude for all of the rich encounters, realizations and ever-deepening perspectives you experienced today. Count your blessings. Inhale deeply and then let it all go in one big breath, surrendering and giving it all up. Breathe into the relaxed, unencumbered feeling enveloping you and the wonderfully rejuvenating, regenerating and restorative sleep awaiting you.

Meditation can involve just about anything that inspires or appeals to your own sensibility. There are formal practices involving mantras, visualizations, resonating tones and focusing on the breath. Another concept of living consciously is to make your daily life and activities, a "living, breathing, walking" meditation. Any activity that puts you "in the zone" – be it gardening, dancing, fishing, writing, family time, pet time, yoga, music, being in nature or simply getting some bodywork therapy – contributes to lightening, softening and opening your heart, mind and body.

> "You should sit in meditation for 20 minutes a day, unless you're too busy; then you should sit for an hour."
> – ANCIENT ZEN WISDOM

ZEN BREATHING MEDITATION: QUIETING THE MIND

This type of meditation uses the breath as a focus of aware-ness. The practice of consciously observing the breath is one of the simplest ways to connect to Spirit. It's what makes this practice so effective. By focusing on the breath, we become less distracted by our chattering, busy minds.

> "If your mind is empty, it is always ready for anything; it is open to everything. In the beginner's mind there are many possibilities; but in the expert's mind there are few."
> – SHUNRYU SUZUKI ROSHI

There are many meditation practices involving the breath, especially when used in conjunction with mantra, counting or imagery. Each of these practices and accompaniments serves as a ground, allowing the mind a focal point (much like mantra) or a place to return each time it wanders. And wander it will. Our mind chatter is accustomed to chiming in, all the time, and needs to be trained that this is "down time." With time and practice, the mind begins to feel more accustomed to the quiet spaciousness and the distracting chatter lessens.

This is the case for those just beginning, as well as more seasoned practitioners. The trick is to continually bring our awareness back to center and follow the breath's inhalation and exhalation, anytime we're aware the mind has wandered. When continually practiced, this meditation will afford greater relaxation, deeper concentration and an overall feeling of peaceful contentment.

"Meditation is not a way of making your mind quiet,
it is a way of entering into the quiet that is already there."
– DEEPAK CHOPRA

ZEN BREATHING MEDITATION TECHNIQUE: COUNTING THE BREATH

- Sit in a comfortable position with the spine straight and head inclined slightly forward.

- Gently close your eyes and take a few deep, natural breaths through your nose.

- Allow your breath to slowly and quietly establish a rhythm without trying to influence it.

- When you're ready to begin, count "one" to yourself on the out-breath.

- Deeply inhale and on the next exhalation, count "two."

- Next out-breath count "three" and continue up to "five."

- Once you reach "five." you've completed the first cycle and should begin a new "five-count" cycle.

"Breath is the bridge that connects life to consciousness;
that unites your body to your thoughts."
– THICH NHAT HANH

We begin this practice using the five-count technique to have an affirming experience. It also lets you know how focused or distracted your mind is in that moment. When you find yourself easily and steadily progressing through *many* five-count cycles, you can increase to a "10-count" cycle. The higher the number, the easier it is for thoughts to float in and out, causing us to forget that we were even counting. You will know your attention has wandered when you find yourself way past your allotted number count. Usually we are not aware that we've spun out on a mind-chatter tangent, replete with to-do lists, previous replays of conversations, concerns, etc., all swirling around in our head.

When you find this occurring, bring your focus gently back to center and start counting once again on the out-breath. This type of distraction is a common occurrence, especially in the beginning – until the mind becomes entrained to steadfastly observe the breath without wandering.

> "As you live deeper in the heart, the mirror
> gets clearer and clearer."
> – RUMI

With practice, you will find yourself experiencing a very deep state of mental relaxation and rejuvenation in a surprisingly short period of time. This practice will prove to be an important asset in maintaining a relaxed, harmonious sense of well-being. Conscious awareness of breath allows us to connect with Spirit.

INVERSION THERAPY
INVERTED POSTURES

Inversion is the simple act of having your feet elevated higher than your head or heart. By reversing gravity, inversion therapy increases blood flow and circulation throughout the body and is considered highly beneficial. It can be as easy as having your feet elevated while watching TV, lying on the floor with a pillow under your feet or even raising your legs up against the wall for 10-15 minutes. For decades, I have personally slept with a small, travel-size pillow under the foot of my mattress, or had risers put under the foot of my bed. I find it has helped give me a rosier complexion, reduced spider veins on my feet and legs, and supported my brain to feel more engaged upon wakening.

With a very little investment of time, energy or exertion, inversion therapy delivers a tremendous amount of value.

Here are some of the recognized benefits of having your feet elevated:

- *Promotes a healthy, glowing complexion.* The increased blood flow to the face provides the facial capillaries with nutrient-rich oxygen, giving the skin a healthy, natural glow.

- *Helps nourish the brain and body with improved blood supply.* The brain accounts for a very small percentage of our body's weight, but uses anywhere from 20-25 percent of the body's oxygen and energy supply. The body and brain both depend on increased oxygen for cell rejuvenation and boosting brain function. Since the blood carries oxygen, improved circulation is key.

- *Improves lymph drainage and fortifies immunity.* Any form of inversion therapy will help stimulate lymphatic cleansing, which moves, clears and drains any toxins from our tissues. With the lymphatic system cleansed, our immune system functions more efficiently and effectively.

- *Helps to calm the nervous system, producing feelings of relaxation, calmness and balance.* It does this by stimulating the production of melatonin and serotonin, which are hormones that assist in relaxing muscle tension, leaving us feeling more calm and relaxed.

"Happiness is when what you think,
what you say and what you do are in Harmony."
— MAHATMA GANDHI

RESTORATIVE BODY/MIND ALIGNMENTS

Yoga, Tai Chi and Qigong are a few of the restorative and regenerative practices we can do for balancing the body and mind. They can be wonderfully relaxing or dynamically stimulating experiences, depending on the form, style or practice used. They all involve the gentle stretching of muscles, breathing exercises, mental concentration and relaxation techniques. These in turn help foster a more awakened state of awareness in our body, mind and emotions, and in how we move through the world.

Our thoughts are extremely powerful.
Our life is a direct reflection of the thoughts,
beliefs and visions we once held.

YOGA: The word yoga comes from the Sanskrit word, Yuj, meaning to yoke, to join or unite. Yoga cultivates the union of the body, mind and spirit, an experience we can realize through the practice of body postures and alignment, breathing exercises, internal relaxation techniques and meditation.

> "Yoga is the journey of the self, through the self,
> to the self."
> – THE BHAGAVAD GITA

There are many schools or forms of Yoga practice. Here are a few of the ones that I'm familiar with:

- **Ashtanga:** One of the oldest forms of yoga, Ashtanga Yoga is an invigorating, rigorous form that uses a progressive series of focused body postures, combined with synchronized breathing techniques. Think of traditional Ashtanga as the Zen form of yoga. You flow from pose to pose with little distraction, following your breath and staying "present" in each moment. Students learn a series of poses and practice at their own pace while the teacher moves around the room giving personalized instruction and guidance. As the breath is synchronized with the postures, a momentum of energy gathers inside the body, generating heat. This intense, internal heat causes impurities to be released through the body's perspiration. With continual practice, one can expect increased flexibility, stamina and strength of the body. Yoga master K. Pattabhi Jois created this form of yoga and established the Ashtanga Yoga Institute in 1948, in Mysore, India.

- **Bikram:** Bikram Yoga, also known as "hot yoga," consists of postures and breathing exercises practiced in a heated room with temperatures around 105 degrees. It is believed that sweating helps move toxins out of the body, allowing a fresh supply of blood and oxygen to circulate while keeping the immune system fortified. Sessions are typically 45 minutes of standing poses and

45 minutes of floor postures. The same sequence of 26 traditional hatha poses, combined with pranayamic breathing exercises, are said to systematically work every part of the body.

This can be a wonderfully effective practice in the colder weather or if you're experiencing any Yin symptoms of dampness in the body. Practicing yoga in a heated room is also believed to help initiate deeper stretches, while also preventing muscular injury. Bikram Choudhury of Calcutta, India, first introduced this system to the United States in 1971. The overall objective of this practice is to create a fit body and an attentive mind, allowing the physical self to unify with the spiritual self.

- **Hatha:** Hatha Yoga is the most commonly associated form in the West. Traditional Hatha Yoga includes physical postures, mental disciplines, purification procedures, breathing exercises and meditation. On the physical level, postures are held for a certain period of time, increasing as you become more practiced. It is believed that the longer the poses are held, the more beneficial to the body and mind. Beginning Hatha Yoga classes prescribe a slower pace and simple breathing exercises, suited for young and old alike. More advanced classes engage in the deeper rigors of form and application, with greater benefit and well-being to the practitioner. The Hindu sage, Yogi Swatmarama, first introduced the practice of Hatha Yoga in the 15th century in India.

"The study of asana is not about mastering posture.
It's about using posture to understand and
transform yourself."
– B.K.S. IYENGAR

- **Iyengar:** Iyengar is one of the oldest forms of Hatha
  Yoga, and involves different types of therapeutic yoga
  positions using props and supports such as straps,
  chairs, blocks and blankets to help accommodate any
  special needs such as injuries or structural imbalances.
  These props help you to improve your form and
  alignment with each posture. Poses are typically held
  longer than in other schools of yoga, so that you can
  pay close attention to the precise muscular and skeletal
  alignment this system demands. As with other forms
  of yoga, Iyengar focuses on the integration of the body
  and mind, regardless of age, proficiency or health.
  B.K.S. Iyengar first introduced his personalized system
  of yoga to the United States in 1956.

"Yoga does not just change the way we see things,
it transforms the person who sees."
– B.K.S. IYENGAR

- **Kundalini:** Kundalini Yoga is considered "the yoga of
  awareness" and tends to be one of the more spiritual
  styles of yoga. This practice is intended to awaken the
  Kundalini "serpent" energy, coiled at the base of the
  spine. This awakening is enabled through the practice
  of certain yoga postures and movement, dynamic
  breathing techniques, and chanting and meditating on

mantras such as "Sat Nam" (translated "I am truth"). As our Kundalini energy becomes unblocked, released and activated, there's a personal transformation within our physical, emotional and mental well-being. Yogi Bhajan founded Kundalini Yoga in the United States in 1969.

"The purpose of training is to tighten the slack, toughen the body and polish the spirit."
– MORIHEI UESHIBA

TAI CHI: (pronounced ty-chee). Tai Chi is a multifaceted practice combining yoga-like movements, meditation, regulated breathing and a series of slow, continual fluid movements of the entire body. The idea is to use your posture, movement, breath and mind to adjust or correct any energetic imbalances or blockages in the body. This can be accomplished by cultivating and increasing the circulation of blood, vital Chi flow and energies throughout the body. This has a tranquilizing effect upon the central nervous system, causing the mind to become clear and relaxed, and the body to feel balanced and stable – resulting in improved muscle strength, coordination and flexibility.

"When you cultivate balance and harmony within yourself or the world, that is Tai Chi. When you work and play with the essence and energy of life...for healing, clarity and inner peace, that is Qigong."
– ROGER JAHNKE, OMD

QI GONG: (pronounced chee-gong) is a philosophical system of cultivating and enhancing energy to maintain or restore balance and harmony within the mind and body. It is a highly effective form of "preventative and restorative health care" that integrates physical postures, breathing techniques and focused intention. The physical postures assist in circulating Chi throughout the body to reduce blockages, deficiencies, congestion and stagnation. The breathing exercises induce a relaxed state of meditation. With focused intention on the breath, the mind moves into a state of clarity and harmonious equilibrium. These combined therapeutic practices assist in reestablishing, maintaining and enhancing body-mind equilibrium, while improving immunity, reducing stress, deepening sleep and increasing strength, coordination, vitality and stamina.

"The most powerful tool you have to change your brain and your health, is your fork."

~ MARK HYMAN MD

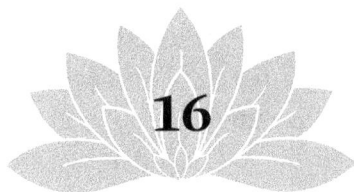

16

Dining Out

During the earlier days of my "vegetarian journey," I can recall dining out with my friends, who ate "normally," and sensing the unspoken, collective-groan when it came time for me to order. Did I really need to ask our waitperson *all* those questions before ordering? Well, at the time I certainly thought I did. I mean, how do you find out what's in your food if you don't ask? As time went on, I thankfully became more refined with my "delivery tone and timbre" when asking questions or voicing concerns. I also got better at flushing out the more acceptable options on just about any menu, irrespective of whether the restaurant served the finest cuisine or was a "mainstream" franchise. Fortunately, I no longer felt the need to bring out the old staccato-fire inquiry about white flour, white sugar, eggs, dairy, MSG or possible meat or meat by-products. What a relief – especially to my fellow dining companions!

My preference has always been to choose the best and most healthful options available, and that is still true for me. However, in looking back, I realize my priorities have shifted and softened over the years when it comes to dining out.

Meaning that, while I still choose the most "preferential" foods for myself, dining out is also about the social enjoyment of being with friends and family. At this point, that seems to take precedent over needing to know a meal's *precise* ingredients. For example, when going out for breakfast, I may find that a restaurant offers buckwheat or whole-grain pancakes, which is great. Am I sure the ingredients are 100 percent whole-grain and have no dairy or eggs? Absolutely not, and that's really OK with me.

You've got to pick and choose where you're going to put your focus, while also covering the things that matter. For me, that has to do with all things meat. Having meat derivatives in my food is simply not an option for me. Because it *is* important to me, I will always ask whether a meal is vegetarian, rather than assume it is – even when it sounds that way. Not much different than someone having a food allergy and making sure that a specific ingredient does not end up in his or her food.

> *Never assume a dish is vegetarian, even if it sounds that way. Many restaurants commonly add chicken broth or beef flavoring to their vegetable-sounding side dishes, soups and sauces.*

The easiest way to implement your dietary preferences when dining out is to communicate clearly and kindly with your server. Are you vegetarian, but eat fish? How about eggs or dairy? What about gluten? If you are a strict vegetarian, you'll want to ask about any meat-based extracts or stock that might be in soups, sauces and veggie-sounding dishes.

The finer restaurants typically have a good assortment of veggies, which are often the side dishes to their main meat entrees. If you're a vegetarian, you'll want to ask if the veggies have been cooked along with the accompanying meat broth, which is a very common practice. Most waiters *do not* know, unless they themselves are practicing vegetarians. They are usually very willing, however, to check with the chef.

If you're trying to stay as gluten-free as possible, let your waiter know. Ask what they might offer in the way of gluten-free substitutions or items. These days, there's an increasing awareness among restaurants to educate their staff, as well as offer gluten-free alternatives. Sometimes your server will assume you have an allergy to wheat, and let you know what other entrees contain wheat. Good to know, even if this may simply be your "preference." Be aware that most of the gluten-free alternatives offered in restaurants tend to be of the *refined* white rice nature. Some of the more trendy restaurants now offer gluten-free products using brown rice, tapioca, coconut or buckwheat flours. You can always ask about the type of replacement flour used.

Perhaps you've entertained the possibility of cutting down on your meat consumption for one meal a day, or possibly one day per week. You might find it easier than imagined, especially with all the veggie-alternatives available. The body does not require animal protein at every meal. In fact, research has shown that a predominantly plant-based diet is not only sufficiently nourishing, but also satisfying as well.

These days, most restaurants offer plenty of meat-free selections along with their usual fare. I'm generally able to find something that will satisfy me at almost any establishment. It's a fairly easy proposition once you familiarize yourself with the options.

HERE ARE SOME POSSIBILITIES

Meat-Free Options and Selections:

- *Italian restaurants:* Eggplant Parmesan, rice or spelt pasta with sautéed veggies in marinara sauce. Vegetable pizza, with gluten-free or whole-grain crust. Mixed vegetable salad with avocado, lemon, Parmesan and olives.

- *Indian restaurants:* Dahl, (spicy lentil soup) samosas, (turnovers) chapattis, papadom (garbanzo-flour crisps), Basmati rice, spinach-paneer, vegetable rice biryani, spinach pakora and vegetable curries.

- *Japanese restaurants:* Edamame, vegetarian nori rolls, brown rice, spring rolls and miso soup. For vegetarians, ask for dishes/soups without oyster sauce and Bonita fish flakes. Same with vegetable tempura – is it fried in the same oil that is used for battered fish?

  Most Japanese and Chinese restaurants offer what they call "wheat meat." For gluten-free folks, this is an absolute no-no. This product is actually vital wheat-gluten, derived from the protein found in wheat. Also known as "seitan," it is commonly found in frozen "veggie meat" products such as *veggie sausage, ribs, bacon, burgers* and *chicken.*

- *Mexican:* Vegetarían fajitas, tacos, enchiladas, tamales, quesadillas, tostadas, burritos, nachos, guacamole, salsa, black or pinto beans and Posole.

- *American restaurants:* The old standbys: Baked potato, salad, steamed or sautéed veggies, minestrone-veggie soup and the ever popular veggie burger.

- *Middle Eastern restaurants:* Falafels, lentil soup, vegetable stew, pita bread, hummus, baba ghanoush, tabouli and couscous.

- *Thai restaurants:* Thai yellow and red curries, lettuce wraps, Pad Thai noodles, veggies and tofu, vegetable spring rolls, green-papaya salad, Thai corn-cakes or fritters, Tom Yum soup (clear broth, spicy), Tom Kha soup (coconut milk base) and mixed green salad. As with Japanese restaurants, ask about oyster sauce in soups, salads and sauces.

- *Chinese restaurants:* Steamed or sautéed vegetables with tofu, cashew chow mein, veggie soups, mixed mushroom sauté, jasmine rice, egg and rice noodles, veggie eggrolls and spring rolls. Ask about MSG (yes, it is still used) and if any fish or oyster sauce is used. Sometimes, I will simply request that no oyster sauce be used in my dish – as opposed to asking.

- *California cuisine.* Tapas style, veggie appetizers. Mixed greens, baby beet salads, grilled vegetables, sautéed kale, collards, leafy greens, wild rice, vegetarian soups, lettuce wraps and boutique fries. (Check out the oil used in frying. Is it is the same oil used for frying battered fish?) Vegetarian pizza. Artichoke/spinach dips, with raw veggies or crostinis. Balsamic salad with nuts, cheese or avocado.

- *Veggie Grill Franchise.* Veggie Grill is a vegan restaurant chain that operates 26+ franchises throughout Southern California, Oregon and Washington. The chain menu offers only plant-based food, with no meat, dairy, eggs, cholesterol, animal fat or trans fat.

Check to see if there are similar kinds of health-oriented restaurant chains in your area.

Part Five
Food Trends, Product Labeling and Consumer Rights

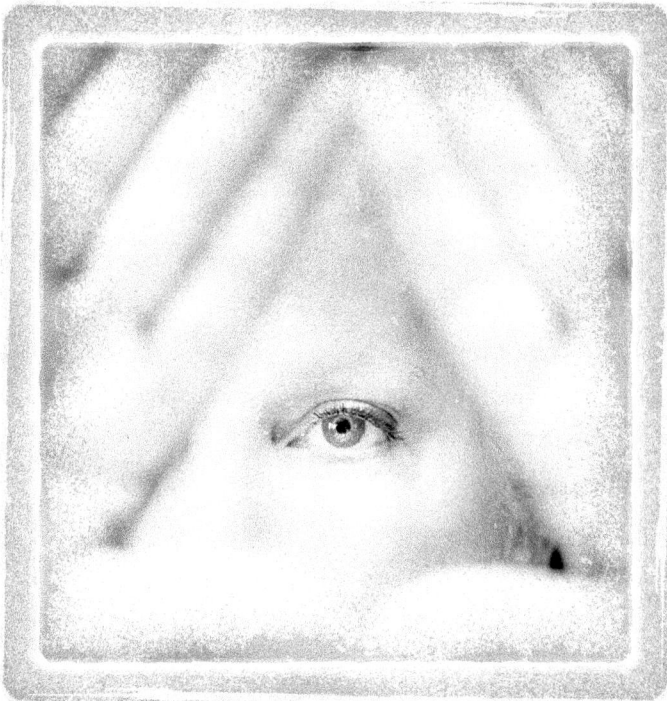

"Clouds gone, the mountain appears."

~ ZEN PROVERB

17

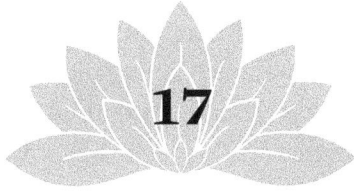

How Do I Know If I'm Gluten Sensitive?

Gluten, as the name implies, is a gluey protein that is present in certain grains. It is especially present in wheat, rye and barley, and to a lesser degree in grains such as spelt, semolina, triticale, couscous, Bulgur and graham flour. Gluten intolerance occurs when there's an inability or difficulty in digesting the grain's gluten proteins. And, while not considered an allergy, there's a broad spectrum of bodily responses to these undigested gluten proteins. Symptoms can range anywhere from mild gluten sensitivity, where the undigested gluten proteins cause gas and bloating, to full blown Celiac, a digestive and autoimmune disorder.

Typically how this works is that the immune system is designed to protect the body from foreign invaders. In the case of those with gluten-intolerance, the immune system recognizes gluten as a foreign invader, much like it would bacteria, and creates antibodies to attack it. These antibodies cause the intestinal lining to become inflamed, damaging the tiny hair-like filaments (villi) that are responsible for absorbing nutrients. When we're not able to absorb nutrients properly, we become deficient and malnourished. This can lead to a host of maladies such as chronic fatigue, food allergies, food sensitivities, skin rashes and nutritional deficiencies. It's important to note that while gluten certainly can contribute toward these symptoms, it isn't *always* the sole culprit. An overload of processed sugar, chemicals, alcohol, antibiotics and environmental toxins can also produce similar responses in the body.

Now, the interesting fact is that all grains contain gluten, even the "gluten-free" ones such as brown rice. It's often times not the gluten per se that people react to, but the specific gluten *proteins* found in grain, such as gliadin and glutenin, that cause indigestibility and sensitivity.

Not too long ago, I had a revelation of sorts about this very subject. I had noticed the appearance of a light, itchy rash on the inside of my forearms and tops of my thighs. I found it curious, because the same rash had also appeared a couple of times before, in precisely the same places, and I hadn't yet figured out the cause. I was simply aware that the rash was itchy and kind of hot, like a form of Yang heat exiting my body. Knowing that one of the ways the body rids itself of offensive or toxic substances is via the lymph system and skin, I realized there was a good chance that this rash was somehow food related. Question was, which food?

For many years, my diet has mostly been oriented toward eating veggies, fruits, plant-based proteins and natural fats – with very little grain. As a result, I was somewhat ambivalent when it came to all of the "gluten-free" products now populating the grocery store shelves. Seemed like everything had a "gluten-free" label plastered across the front. It was the new marketing "catch-phrase" much like all the previous advertising slogans of "natural," "low-fat," "no-MSG," "low-cal," "reduced sugar" or "no trans-fat."

I rarely ate refined wheat-flour products such as bread, muffins, pancakes or pasta that contained gluten – or so I thought. I would have the occasional cooked whole grain during the colder winter months, and maybe some whole grain chips or crackers as a snack, but for the most part, grains played a very marginal role in my daily diet.

I did, however, include a few tasty, frozen, veggie-meat products on occasion made from vital wheat gluten. I hadn't really thought a lot about it. They seemed relatively clean with no obvious offending ingredients, nor animal derivatives, so, away I ate. Interesting thing was, when I did consume these seasoned veggie-meats, I would typically have them for days in a row, until the package was finished. Now, for someone whose body is not used to it, that's a fair amount of wheat gluten to be taking in, relatively speaking. The more I looked into this, the more I suspected a connection between the amount of gluten I was consuming, and the appearance of my rash. I decided to do a little experiment, and eliminate all gluten products from my diet for a number of months and see what happened.

As was typical, I never saw any kind of rash during that time. I then introduced the gluten veggie-meat and ate it for my usual, few days in succession. Within a week and a half time period: There. It. Was. The same light rash in the same location. Very telling. I do believe that in my case, this was more related to the *amount* of vital wheat gluten I was taking in succession, as opposed to having it only on occasion. To this day, I've not experienced any noticeable reaction or sensitivity to whole-wheat products (organic and sprouted) or vital wheat gluten for that matter, when I partake with intuitive discretion and moderation.

Signs of Glucose sensitivity or intolerance:

- Digestive issues
- Problems absorbing nutrients, due to intestinal inflammatory response
- Chronic fatigue due to lack of nutrient absorption
- Brain fog and difficulty concentrating
- Low immunity
- Skin rashes and eczema-like bumpy skin patches
- Inflammatory response causing joint pain and headaches
- Mood swings due to hormonal imbalances

Just a little heads up as you start exploring the wide variety of gluten-free products available: Many of them are cleverly marketed as natural, but are really no better than their empty, filler-food predecessors. Manufacturers simply remove the "offending" wheat flour, and replace it most commonly with refined rice flour. Frequently used substitutions also include processed cornstarch, tapioca starch, potato starch and guar gum. A preferred choice would be gluten-free products made with whole grain, gluten-free flours such as buckwheat or brown-rice flour or grain-free flours such as coconut, almond or hazelnut flours.

Says Dr. William Davis, MD, author of the popular book, *Wheat Belly,* "Every day, over 200 million Americans consume food products made of wheat. As a result, over 100 million of them experience some form of adverse health effect, ranging from minor rashes and high blood sugar to unattractive stomach bulges." Davis refers to these stomachs, as "wheat bellies." He attributes this to the wheat protein called gliadin, found in the newer strains of hybrid wheat.[10] He believes that gliadin acts as an opiate to the brain, stimulating our appetite. It's his conclusion that "wheat is the single largest contributor to our nation's obesity epidemic, and its elimination in the American diet, is key, to dramatic weight loss and optimal health."[11]

This has much to do with the fact that our modern wheat is nothing like the wheat of our ancestors. During the Industrial Revolution, there came technologies to improve agricultural efficiency and output, which in turn, changed how we grew and processed cereal grain crops. Stone-ground milling was now replaced with mechanical milling. This kind of milling pulverized and ground the wheat into nutrient-stripped, barren white flour that wasn't as prone to rancidity. One of the upsides of this refined, white flour was that it produced a much lighter and fluffier bakery product – one for which we quickly developed a taste and a preference.

Next came newer and more "progressive" chemical-applications and biotechnology. This experimental technology took the form of chemical-laden fertilizers, herbicides, fungicides and insecticides, which presumably made wheat crops more resistant to insects, weeds, drought and blight. This was done all in the name of larger crop production and the resultant increases in revenue. The problem was, there was very little thought given to the health and welfare of the unsuspecting consumer – who happened to be ingesting those potentially noxious, biotech chemical-constituents.

David Perlmutter, MD, author of the book, *Grain Brain*, believes that these newer, aggressive forms of hybridization created grains with up to 40 times the amount of gluten than those of prior decades. Americans cannot process the gluten from these new hybridized grains.

There is a growing movement toward the ancient heritage wheats, such as einkorn, spelt and emmer, that have lower gluten content, offering many folks a respite from the typical symptoms and sensitivity from modern wheat. There's also an heirloom variety of wheat called Turkey Red Wheat, originally from the Ukraine, that is gaining popularity for its great baking qualities and superb flavor.

18

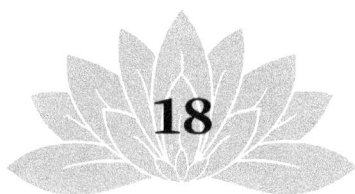

No Fat, Low Fat, Whole Fat? Is Fat Ever Good?

When it came to the subject of dietary fat, I was in relatively foreign territory. Truth was, I'd never really thought too much about the subject. I knew that the body used fat as fuel, but that was about it. Being a vegetarian, I figured that as long as I ate enough nuts, seeds and avocado, naturally processed green olives, salad dressings, sesame and olive oils, and the occasional bit of cultured dairy, I'd be OK, which proved correct.

Most of the negative commentary I'd heard about fats had to do with saturated animal fats, which played a very small role in my diet. I'd occasionally have some cultured dairy, such as yogurt, kefir or sour cream. I was also comfortable having some shaved Parmesan or butter on my veggies or potato when dining out. While fats were not a major focus for me, I did observe the widespread trend toward "all things low fat."

It appeared that many of the prevalent medical conditions (obesity, high cholesterol and congestive heart disease) had to do with an excess of saturated fat clogging up arteries and organs, and raising cholesterol levels. These issues seemed to arise especially when too much fat was combined with a sedentary lifestyle. Typically the advice from the medical profession was a simple, "cut down on animal fat consumption." OK, but what did that mean to the average person and how were they supposed to actually incorporate this "cutting down on fat?"

Generally, doctors are not trained in the field of holistic health and nutrition, so the simplest suggestion was to seek out reduced fat or no-fat foods. It was the late 1980s and the ever-opportunistic food industry answered the "call" for reduced-fat foods by simply replacing saturated animal fats in food products with unsaturated vegetable oil.

However, it really wasn't as simple as just exchanging out the fat for the oil. The suitable replacement had to replicate the accustomed "palatability," which included the old familiar texture, stability, flavor and sweetness that consumers were used to. Cue in the industry's food scientists to create and combine hydrogenated oils, artificial flavoring, emulsifiers, stabilizers, texture-agents, chemical sweeteners and additional salt, to replicate comparable tastes and textures.

Before you knew it, the cleverly targeted advertising campaigns had us believing that these wonderful "low-fat" foods were akin to "health foods." Soon, we were all convinced that reduced-fat or low-fat items were *the* way to go, for two very good reasons: they were supposedly good for us *and* they would not make us fat. Was this true? Well, we certainly had it on good authority. So, with our ever-adaptable minds and nature, we came to believe that by consuming these new "healthy fat" alternatives, we were proactively contributing to our good health and our families.

These "healthfully" marketed foods now took the form of prepackaged "convenience" foods, such as pastas, dips, faux dairy products, frozen meals, soups, snack foods, fast foods and sugary treats. Funny thing was, saturated (animal) fat consumption did go down, but due to the high caloric, artificial content of these reduced-fat foods, people continued to pile on the pounds.

The challenge with such a diet is that the body does not do well with processing these nutrient-poor, faux-fat, sugary foods, and instead ends up storing them as fat. Yep, storing them as fat, and not the good kind of fat that our body actually needs to operate efficiently. So, contrary to popular opinion that a low-fat diet could and would reduce obesity, hypertension, atherosclerosis and heart attacks – there was instead, a notable escalation of these conditions.

> *The challenge with a reduced-fat diet is that the body does not know how to process these nutrient-poor, faux fat substitutes, and they end up being stored as fat.*

So, what do you do with this "fat" information, especially if you want to get a handle on maintaining a healthier, leaner body? Well, if you are already eating a balanced whole-foods diet or moving toward one, I can tell you that eating with awareness, being conscious of portions, expanding veggie and clean protein intake and moving your body a bit more, will absolutely do wonders for you.

When foods are eaten in their most natural, whole state, the way nature intended, our bodies instinctively know how to process the naturally occurring blend of nutrients, fats, proteins and sugar. If you desire a dairy product, then it's best to have it in its natural, whole-milk form. Once the fat is reduced or removed, the original balanced chemistry becomes altered. It's the same with eggs. Eat an egg whole, rather than separating the yolk from the whites. Nature has included a precise amount of lecithin in the yolk to handle the natural fat. If possible, go with whole-milk yogurt, rather than the low-fat versions. Use natural butter, rather than margarine.

Not surprisingly, when it comes to fats, you've got to pay attention to the type of fat *and* the amount you're ingesting. You will know, and intuit what the "correct" balance is for you. Our body is brilliant that way, especially the more you tune in. Consuming smaller portions, and eating slower and more consciously – will go a long way toward supporting a harmoniously balanced body and mind. The simplest caveat to remember is that the healthiest foods tend to be the least processed.

If you've ever wondered what the difference is between saturated, poly-unsaturated and mono-unsaturated fatty acids, and how they fit into a healthfully balanced diet, here's a basic overview from my perspective.

SATURATED FATS

I think of saturated fats as "sat-fats," meaning they remain solid or semi-solid when they sit out. These are the densest of fats. Think of lard, butter and coconut oil. Sat-fats are also the least prone to rancidity. While these types of fat add flavor and easily handle higher cooking temperatures, a little goes a long way. This is especially so if your diet is already high in meat and dairy products, as sat-fats are primarily found in red meat, poultry, cheese, eggs, cream and butter.

Plant based sources of sat-fats include oils from coconut and red palm. Moderation is the key word when it comes to sat-fats. A peppering of these high fat foods seems to work well for most, and significantly well when combined with a high amount of nutrient rich, antioxidant, leafy greens, including kale, collards, chard, arugula and cilantro.

Sat-fats are the least prone to rancidity and can handle the highest cooking temperatures.

MONO-UNSATURATED AND POLY-UNSATURATED FATS

Mono-unsaturated and poly-unsaturated fats are, as their name implies, un-saturated, meaning they remain liquid in oil form sitting at room temperature. You'll want to get the majority of your fats from these two categories. The biggest challenge with these oils, particularly the poly-oils, (whether in seed, nut or extracted oil form) is their high susceptibility toward rancidity, especially when *exposed* to light, heat or air. Light. Heat. Air. Which pretty much guarantees rancidity in a few short months, unless they are kept in the refrigerator, where I've taken to storing them.

Sat-Fats	Mono-Fats	Poly-Fats	Trans-Fats
Meats	Olive Oil	Sunflower Oil	Hydrogenated Oils, Partially Hydrogenated Oils
Poultry	Avocados	Safflower Oil	Pastries, Desserts, Pies, Donuts
Cheeses	Canola Oil	Flaxseed Oil	Fried, Breaded Foods
Eggs	Almonds	Chia, Hemp	Snack Foods, Chips
Butter	Peanut Oil	Soy Oil	Veg. Shortening
Ghee	Hazelnuts	Pumpkin Seeds	Stick Margarine
Lard	Sesame Oil	Fatty Fish – salmon, mackerel, tuna, trout, sardines, anchovy	Dips, Spreads, Salad Dressings
Coconut Oil	Pecans	Tempeh, Tofu, Edamame	Candy Bars
Palm Oil	Macadamias	Walnuts	
Cocoa Butter	High Oleic Oils	Spirulina	

When exposed to heat, light and air, Mono and Poly-oils are most susceptible to rancidity – and therefore best stored in the refrigerator.

MONO-UNSATURATED FATS

Mono-fats are typically considered the healthiest of fats, because they lower the "undesirous" cholesterol and raise the "good" cholesterol. They are especially helpful in reducing inflammation and assisting in the regulation of insulin and blood sugar levels. These healthy mono-fats are contained in olives, avocados, almonds, hazelnuts, sesame and pecans. The more recently developed plant-strains of high-oleic sunflower and safflower oils now have a higher ratio of healthy mono-fats than before, making them more stable and less prone to rancidity.

Mono-oils are best suited for light cooking, sautéing and salad dressings.

POLY-UNSATURATED FATS
(The Essential Fatty Acids)

Poly-fats are known as the essential fatty acids, because our body is not able to create them and must get them from food sources. Essential fatty acids, especially the Omega-3s, are exceptionally beneficial to our bodies. They've been found to strengthen immunity, fight inflammation, increase brain and neurological function, lower triglycerides and support adrenal and thyroid activity. I personally have found a marked improvement in my brain's alertness, clarity and responsiveness, since taking them.

Along with protecting and fortifying our brain and cell walls, fats – especially the very important Omega-3 fatty acids – help our brain-messaging system and nervous system run smoothly and efficiently.

These Poly essential fatty acids are found in the seed oils of flax, chia, hemp and pumpkin. Spirulina, edamame, tempeh and walnuts are also considered rich sources. The highest marine sources tend to be salmon, tuna, trout, mackerel, sardine, anchovy, herring, krill and marine micro-algae. Micro-algae are the microscopic algae that marine fish consume to produce Omega-3s. The Omega-3 fish oils have been found very assistive in "roto-rooting" out the animal sat-fats lining many a clogged artery.

Poly-oils are best consumed cold and unheated, as in salad dressings, rather than used in cooking. Only when Poly-oils are in their high-oleic form should they be used for cooking.

Poly-oils are best stored in the refrigerator or a cool, dark space. Think of the times you've checked on a bottle of oil at home, only to find it rancid. I certainly have. I personally keep all my oils in the fridge these days, for the simple reason that I use them very sporadically – and I find they last longer without going rancid.

It's always a good rule of thumb to periodically check the aroma and expiration date of your household oils due to the high rancidity factor.

REFINED OILS

It's best to stay away from any conventionally extracted oils that use high heat and the toxic, petro-chemical solvent, hexane. These oils are often labeled as "refined" oils. Look for the oils that are labeled expeller-pressed, cold-pressed and hexane-free. The healthiest method of extraction is expeller-pressed and cold-pressed. These methods are the best at preserving the flavor, aroma and nutrients, without using high-heat or toxic chemical processing.

HYDROGENATED OILS (TRANS FAT)

It is also best to stay away from any food that lists "hydrogenated" or even "partially hydrogenated" oil in its ingredients. Hydrogenated Oil is a Trans-Fat. As I described in Chapter 6, this process extracts the naturally occurring oil from corn, soybean, palm or coconut and puts it under severe heat and pressure, while adding chemical catalysts. This causes a transformation in the oil's molecular structure, changing the liquid texture of the oil into a thicker, semi-solid or solid form, such as Crisco or margarine.

This process was originally created to address the problem of rancidity within baked goods, snack foods, fried foods, non-dairy creamers and margarine-type spreads. The challenge with this coagulated greasy trans-fat is that it thickens the blood's viscosity, causing it to coat and clog the arteries and blood vessels. This then causes additional strain on the heart to pump this thickened, sludgy blood throughout the body. Not a good thing.

The first three types of fat cited (Sat, Mono and Poly) are extremely important for the brain and nerve receptors to communicate effectively and efficiently with the body. Fats are also very important in boosting the immune system, improving vitamin and mineral utilization, creating healthier, supple skin, producing and regulating hormones, assisting with liver function, promoting nutrient absorption and detoxification – and surprisingly – helping us maintain a desirable weight.

19

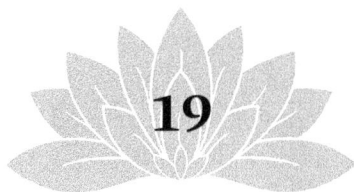

Caffeine and Adrenal Fatigue

My earliest recollections regarding coffee were mostly of my Mom and Grandmother brewing a pot in the morning. During high school, my friends and I readily drank sodas (Coca-Cola, Pepsi, Dr Pepper and Mountain Dew) and I'm sure we never gave a moment's thought to any of the soda's ingredients. Certainly not the caffeine content – which I now realize was quite considerable. It wasn't until I got into natural foods and became more label conscious, that I was apprised of the varying levels of caffeine found in food, beverages and pills. I had no idea.

While I would occasionally try a sip or two of coffee, I mostly found it bitter, with very little upside. As a result, it never became a preferred ritual for me. Decades later, I would find myself sitting at an outdoor café somewhere in Europe, Asia or Mexico, taking in the cultural sights around me, and yes, actually sipping an espresso. And while it still tasted bitter, a bit of honey and cream would go a long way to making it reasonably palatable. (Alternative milks were non-existent at this time.) More than the taste however, was the wonderful feeling of being immersed in the local culture and experiencing a heightened sense of awareness in my mind and body. This was really the *first* time I experienced the pleasurable "buzz" associated with caffeine, and understood why it was such a desirable ritual (or addiction) for so many.

To this day, I still find it to be a wonderful energetic enhancement. And that's precisely how I think about it. I use it before a workout, as a mood-booster or before anything cerebral – and of course, anytime I travel.

While I've come to appreciate caffeine's wonderfully "boosting" attributes, I've also experienced the times when it has had a very exhausting effect on my body and adrenals. It's understandable why caffeine is the preferred drink for so many as a morning "wake-up" and in the afternoon as an effective "pick-me-up" when energy wanes. There is nothing wrong with that unless like me, you begin to experience those times when your body feels dull and drained afterwards. It may only happen occasionally – and that's a good thing. It means your adrenals are still functioning as intended. What it *does* tell you is that your adrenals are becoming fatigued and some corrective action would be prudent.

First, let's take a look at why caffeine affects us the way it does.

HOW CAFFEINE WORKS IN OUR BODIES

Have you ever wondered why or how caffeinated beverages, like coffee, colas, teas or sports drinks give us that desired boost? It has a great deal to do with brain chemistry. One of the reasons we feel more alert, uplifted and more dexterous with caffeine in our system, is that like any other stimulant, it causes an increase in our brain's production of the neurotransmitter dopamine. Dopamine is one of the brain's "elevating" chemical stimulants that promote a feeling of positivity, pleasure, optimism and enjoyment.

Dopamine also triggers those parts of the brain involved with problem solving, motivation and memory. On a physical level, dopamine helps us feel more grounded and "aware" in our body. It also fosters a greater sense of motor control when engaged in physical activity. Yep, when used therapeutically, caffeine is one of the best tonics around – on every level. No wonder we like this stuff.

Another thing caffeine does, is stimulate the brain's communication switchboard. This stimulation increases neuro-firing (neuro=nerve) and neuro-transmitting capabilities – the specific way the brain communicates with the rest of the body. This amplified nerve activity triggers the brain to send a preparatory alert that "something's up" to the adrenal glands. These small glands that sit atop the kidneys then release adrenaline, the flight-or-fight hormone. When adrenaline is released, it signals the liver to release some stored reserves of blood sugar, which is the high-octane fuel needed by the body and brain to handle any potential threat or crisis. In other words, this high-octane fuel speeds up our metabolism, which enables more blood to be pumped throughout the body.

This in turn heightens performance and response time, facilitating the most effective action. This heightened response and accompanying attributes, is what we experience when drinking a good old cup of Joe. We're left with a stimulated mind and invigorated body, prompting us to feel more efficient, effective and responsive in our daily lives. Easy to see why coffee is our "go to" beverage of choice.

WHEN CAFFEINE BECOMES A "TAKE-AWAY"

Whenever a stimulant (or medication) is taken regularly, the body has a tendency to build up a resistance and eventually needs more to achieve the same effect. When greater amounts of caffeine are used and used habitually, there's a constant triggering of adrenal stimulation, prepping us for an "emergency" that never comes. Without a physical discharge or expenditure of this primed, blood sugar-fuel now coursing through our veins, we are left feeling jittery, stressed, anxious and frazzled, with a great likelihood of restlessness or insomnia later on.

Once our adrenaline levels finally taper off, the brain and body experience low blood sugar. The brain is most directly affected, because it does not store blood sugar (fuel) and depends on moment-to-moment blood sugar from food or stored body reserves to function properly. After the "crash," the brain is left fuel-deficient, essentially running on fumes. Without the necessary fuel to power the brain, you can count on exhaustion, brain-fog, headaches and irritability.

Another hormone that's triggered alongside adrenaline during stressful times is cortisol, otherwise known as the "stress hormone." Similar in its response to adrenaline, the brain does not differentiate whether that stress is tension-related, caffeine-generated or involves surviving a "true" emergency. In our earliest ancestral times when famine was common, cortisol was the specific hormone that helped us survive.

Whenever the body senses that reserves are low, or there's less food coming in, it automatically kicks in cortisol to slow down our metabolism. This is so the body can actually survive on less food until we're able to replenish once again. This is the very reason why we *don't* lose weight when we're stressed out, or decrease our food intake (as in dieting), or when we simply replace a meal with a quick and easy caffeinated drink. You'd think by taking in less food and stepping up our pace when we're stressed, we'd lose weight. Not the case. These behaviors trigger *increased* cortisol levels, that actually produce the opposite effect – *that of gaining weight* – especially belly fat. As our body metabolism slows down for survival, surplus fat is transferred from other areas of the body (hips and rump) to the abdomen where cortisol receptors are plentiful.

These days, our most typical stressors tend to be related to financial, work, health and relationship issues. Whatever the cause, the outcome is the same: high levels of cortisol (and adrenaline) constantly being released – and affecting every physiological system in the body. When stress-induced cortisol and adrenaline levels remain elevated, adrenal fatigue sets in, compromising our immune system, causing erratic blood sugar levels, increased moodiness, behavioral outbursts, high blood pressure, premature aging, diminished libido and weight gain – especially abdominal fat.

HOW TO HANDLE CAFFEINE AND STRESS AND STILL REMAIN BALANCED

With the understanding that excess caffeine, sugar and stress all have the same effect on our body, brain and adrenals, our ultimate mission becomes that of stabilizing the erratic rise and fall of blood sugar. That takes some reorienting and readjusting on our part, and a reworking of some of our prior habits and patterning. Once we understand the actual "cause and effect" of these stressors and how they trigger our body chemistry – the more apt we are to make a change. Especially one that is in our best interest.

Here are some helpful ways to make that change and support your adrenals:

First, when it comes to caffeine, studies have shown that the best windows for consumption are *after breakfast*, between 10 a.m. and noon, and in the afternoon slump period, between 2 and 5 p.m. Here is the reason why: These are the times when caffeine *will not* interfere with the natural and helpful cycles of cortisol production in the body. For example, cortisol levels are the highest in the morning, which naturally promotes the feeling of "being awake." Studies have also shown that when people think they've developed a "tolerance" for coffee, it's actually because their morning caffeine has caused cortisol levels to rise unnaturally, which gives the body a false read that cortisol levels are flush. As a result, the body's natural morning production of cortisol decreases, leaving us feeling "less awake" and needing more coffee.[12] And so, while not always convenient, the best solution is to partake of our caffeinated beverages later, during the 10 a.m.-to-noon window. As always – you do the best you can and remember the "*spirit* of the law, rather than the *letter* of the law."

Second, developing healthfully balanced eating habits, such as getting "enough" good quality protein in the morning, especially before that 10 a.m.-to-noon window, will go a long way to help regulate blood sugar. If sugar, stress and caffeine are the things that cause erratic blood sugar, think of protein as the "efficient stabilizer." I tend to make a morning smoothie during the warmer months, using *Garden of Life,* Organic Plant Protein powder, along with *Vibrant Health,* Green Vibrance, an organic superfood powder with nutrients, greens and grasses.

Third, there are specific adaptogen herbs and supplements that can be especially helpful.

Investigate on your own and see which ones resonate with you:

- *Siberian ginseng* reduces fatigue and helps treat and repair damaged proteins during times of intense stress and physical demand.

- *Omega-3 fatty acids* reduce inflammation and assist with adrenal resiliency.

- *Ashwagandha* helps regulate the body's cortisol levels, decrease anxiety, enhance immune function and improve sleep.

- *D-Ribose* helps deliver energy-rich blood to ATP-depleted muscles and assists with fatigue, exhaustion and muscle pain. (ATP is the biochemical energy used to power the movement of contraction in working muscles)

- *Magnesium* helps relieve stress and relaxes the muscles and body.

- *Astragalus root* is a great Chi tonic – enhancing body energy, boosting immunity and building stamina and vitality.

- *Cordyceps mushroom* helps to stabilize blood sugar levels and strengthen the immune system. As a stimulant, it is used to increase energy and enhance stamina.

- *Rhodiola* assists in balancing blood sugar and protects against stress-related fatigue. It is also known to elevate mood levels and help alleviate depression and anxiety.

- *Licorice root* has been shown helpful in balancing and supporting the adrenal glands, and in restoring normal cortisol levels.

- *Holy Basil (Tulsi)* has been shown effective in counteracting fatigue, boosting immunity and regulating blood sugar, blood pressure and hormone levels.

As an alternative to coffee, adaptogenic teas, such as black tea, green tea or Yerba Mate', have been shown to improve the body's ability to cope with stress, especially adrenal stress. Adaptogens are a unique class of healing plants that help balance, restore and protect the body's physiological functions. They help counteract the adverse effects of stress by enhancing the cells' utilization of oxygen, thus eliminating residual metabolic toxicity, and enhancing our body's own resilience and adaptability. One such adaptogen is L-Theanine, found in black tea and green teas such as Sencha, Gyokuro and Matcha – with Matcha containing the highest amount. L-Theanine has been shown to neutralize the speedy, jagged effects of caffeine without reducing its mind-enhancing, fat-burning features.

Since I tend to use caffeine as an "energetic enhancement," it falls into the medicinal category for me. That means I use it mindfully and somewhat judiciously, as opposed to habitually. My consumption changes often, depending on my circumstances and intuition. Some days I'll have none and other days I may have two cups. On average, it typically translates to one cup a day of espresso, chai or Yerba Mate'. The best way I've found to use caffeine for the utmost benefit is to adjust the amount to fit the circumstance. More often than not, half of the typical amount will do the trick. Plus, as weird as it sounds, when I'm home, I'll throw a few raw pumpkin or sunflower seeds in and actually chew my drink. The seed protein and fat allows my body to handle the caffeine better and feel more balanced. I also make sure to have an equal amount of water afterwards. The water not only dilutes the acidity, but also rehydrates my body from the diuretic effect of the caffeine.

Caffeine Amounts in Food and Beverages[13]

Food or Beverage	Amount	Caffeine Content
COFFEE		
Coffee, generic brewed	8 oz	102-200 mg
Coffee, Starbucks brewed	12 oz (tall)	260 mg
Latte or Cappuccino, Starbucks	12 oz (tall)	75 mg
Expresso, Starbucks	1 oz	75 mg
Expresso, generic	1 oz	30-90 mg
Coffee, generic instant	8 oz	27-173 mg
Coffee, generic decaffeinated	8 oz	3-26 mg
TEA		
Black Tea, brewed	8 oz	25-110 mg (average 45 mg)
Green Tea, brewed	8 oz	10-50 mg (average 20 mg)
Yerba Mate, loose	1-2 Tbsp. 8oz	65–135 mg
White Tea, brewed	8 oz	5-25 mg (average 15 mg)
Oolong Tea, brewed	8 oz	12-60 mg (average 45 mg)
Rooibos Tea, brewed	8 oz	0-0.4 mg
Tazo Chai Tea Latte, Starbucks	12 oz (tall)	70 mg
Nestea Iced Tea	12 oz	26 mg
Snapple Iced Tea	16 oz	42 mg
Lipton Brisk Iced Tea	12 oz	10 mg
SOFT DRINKS		
Coke	12 oz	35 mg
Pepsi	12 oz	38 mg
Jolt Cola	12 oz	72 mg
Mountain Dew	12 oz	54 mg
7-Up	12 oz	o mg
Sprite	12 oz	0 mg
ENERGY DRINKS		
Red Bull	8.3 oz	80 mg
SoBe Essential Energy, berry or orange	8 oz	48 mg
SoBe No Fear	8 oz	83 mg
DESSERTS		
Dark Chocolate	1.45 oz bar	32 mg
Milk Chocolate	1.45 oz bar	11 mg
Coffee Ice Cream or Frozen Yogurt	8 oz	50-60 mg
Hot Chocolate, generic	8 oz	3-13 mg
Chocolate Cake	2.8 oz	36 mg
Chocolate Brownies	1.5 oz	10 mg

Listed below are a few helpful guidelines to consider when exploring ways to balance your caffeine intake and adrenal response:

- *The caffeine content of coffee and tea can vary widely.* You can generally figure a 6 oz. cup of coffee has approximately 100 mg of caffeine. You can count on more, double actually, if you drink from a 12 oz. mug, or get a "small" coffeehouse drink to go. Generally, a maximum of 80-200 mg of caffeine per day is manageable for most. One thing to remember, the darker the roast, the lower the caffeine content, and stronger the taste. An Espresso, single shot, has less caffeine than drip coffee, mainly because we're only ingesting one ounce. Another reason is that drip coffee takes a good few minutes to brew, whereas espresso is "flashed" for 15-20 seconds with highly pressurized water. Black and green teas are lower in caffeine than coffee. A cup of green tea contains less caffeine than black tea.

Caffeine affects our fluid balance and typically has a diuretic effect on the body. It's a good idea to drink equal amounts of water after coffee, tea, soda or energy drinks.

- *Drink more water to rehydrate and to help dilute the acidity.* It is essential to replace water reserves regularly as our human body is more than 72% water. Caffeine is a diuretic, which means it eliminates bodily fluid and can cause dehydration. If you increase your uptake of water, you may also find fewer cravings for soda, coffee or tea.

The human body is more than 72 percent water. Our blood is roughly 83 percent water, lungs 90 percent, skin 80 percent, brain and muscles 75 percent water, and even our bones are about 22 percent water. It is absolutely essential to replenish water reserves regularly, for all biological systems to run smoothly and efficiently.

- *A Macrobiotic practice to counter coffee's acidity is to add a few grains of sea salt per cup.* An *Ayurvedic* solution is to add a pinch of cardamom and ginger to offset the potentially depleting effect coffee has on the nervous system.

"*A donkey carrying Holy books is still a donkey.*"

~ ZEN PROVERB

20

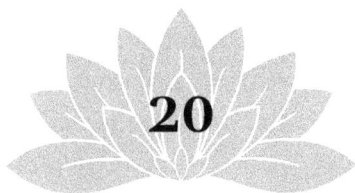

Product Labeling and Consumer Rights

I've been a big label reader, since way back when. This was especially important with all my dietary preferences. I wanted to *know* if a product contained animal by-products, refined sugars, processed grains, chemical additives, flavor-enhancers or preservatives. Fortunately for me, my preferences were by design. For many people with food allergies or food-related medical conditions, eating the wrong foods could prove life threatening.

We may not always have control over the circumstances of our life, but we do have control of what goes in our mouths and bellies.

So, I learned to read food labels diligently and question how meals were prepared at restaurants. This worked well in theory, as long as store-bought items were accurately labeled and waiters were well informed – which wasn't always the case. In my earlier days, I never thought of questioning where the ambiguously labeled "natural" flavors, colors, enzymes, emulsifiers, binders or ingredients came from. Well, consider me now informed. After years of research, I've discovered that several of these "natural" ingredients are actually sourced from animal, fish and insect parts.[14] As someone who would rather *not* ingest these things, I would have preferred knowing that information beforehand.

Did you know that a company can claim a "trade secret" recipe and not be required to list all of those ingredients for fear someone will try to replicate it? For example, the fiercely guarded, "original" trade-secret ingredients for Coca Cola included coca extract, caffeine, sugar, lime juice, vanilla, caramel, orange oil, lemon oil, nutmeg oil, coriander, neroli, cinnamon and a fair amount of alcohol. Who knew?

Wouldn't it be great to have all food ingredients labeled clearly, so we'd actually know what we're eating?

I, like many, assumed there were laws requiring manufacturing companies to *fully disclose* each and every ingredient used in their products. Not the case. This may have been the truth long ago, when *real food* ingredients were used to make real food products. Today, it's a very different story. The Food and Drug Administration (FDA), which regulates fruits, vegetables and most processed foods, doesn't even have an "official" definition for the term, "natural." Advertisers can market their food as "all natural," but that does not in any way, guarantee their products are GMO free. A product can contain dubiously sourced chemicals, flavors, sweeteners and genetically modified foods, and still be labeled as "natural." Makes absolutely *no* sense to me.

The two government agencies, USDA and the FDA, that supposedly are charged with the duty of monitoring and regulating food safety and labeling, do not even recognize a distinction between organic, conventional and genetically engineered foods.

Another disturbing piece of information regarding genetically engineered foods is that there are absolutely *no* requirements made upon the biotech companies that engineer these foods, nor any studies conducted by government agencies concerning consumer safety. Many of the reports that are conducted and published are typically from the very companies (Monsanto, Dupont, Syngenta, Dow) that are producing and supporting the genetically modified foods in the first place. I can't imagine that those reports are without bias. Quite the opposite.

There are astounding amounts of money and political influence put forth by large biotech firms to keep the consumer in the dark. Any incriminating evidence is intentionally kept under wrap – so there is not ever the *requirement* to label and declare a food, seed or practice as genetically modified or engineered. If these genetically modified foods, seeds, sprays and farming practices are truly "safe," then what's the problem with disclosing and labeling GMO products? At least that way, consumers can make their own executive decisions on whether to purchase that product or not.

So, what to do? For me it translates very simply. *I want to know what's in my food.* I want sensible disclosure concerning product ingredients. I want authentic transparency around the food farming practices shown to be unsafe and toxic for humans and the environment. Again, what's the big secret? Even mattresses have to have their contents labeled. Disclosure gives me the power and freedom to make informed decisions concerning myself and my family's food, health and well-being. This power of choice is particularly important for individuals dealing with chemical sensitivities, food allergies, immune-deficiencies, antibiotic resistances and nutritional imbalances.

I do my best to "decode" what labels are describing, but with the ever-changing landscape of labeling laws, compa-nies changing ownership and formulas being altered – I'm often in the dark. Half the time I'm running on instincts and prior knowledge, and the rest of the time, I look for the most reputable brand and go for the products that are labeled with "organically grown" ingredients.

On the topic of reputable brands, it's important to know that the whole topography of natural food companies has changed tremendously over the past couple of decades. Many of the larger "commercial" food companies have bought out the smaller, "boutique" natural food companies. It makes you wonder whether the previous "clean" standards of the boutique companies have been compromised as they became absorbed into the "parent" company's long-standing commercial methods and practices. This is another one of those gray areas.

Here are some of those acquisitions:

- Heinz bought Hain Food Group in 1999 for $100 million.

- Hain/Celestial bought Celestial seasonings in 2000 for $390 million.

- J. M. Smucker bought R.W. Knudsen in 1984 and Santa Cruz Naturals in 1989.

- General Mills bought Muir Glen in 1998, Cascadian Farm in 1999 and Annie's in 2014.

- Kellogg's bought Morningstar ($307 million) in 1999 and Kashi ($33 million) in 2000.

- ConAgra bought Lightlife Foods (Smart Bacon, Smart Deli) in 2000.

- Kraft bought Boca Foods and Balance Bar ($268 million) in 2000.

- Unilever bought Ben & Jerry's in 2000 for $326 million.

- Coca-Cola bought Odwalla in 2001 for $181 million.

- Dean bought White Wave/Silk in 2002 for $189 million.

- Hain/Celestial bought Spectrum Organics in 2006 for $33 million.

- Colgate-Palmolive bought Tom's of Maine in 2006 for $100 million.

- Pepsi bought Naked Juice in 2006 for about $450 million.

- Hershey's bought Dagoba Chocolate in 2006.

- Clorox bought Burt's Bees in 2007 for $913 million.

- Coca-Cola bought Energy Brands (Smart Water) in 2007 for $4.2 billion.

- Kellogg bought Bear Naked in 2007 for $122 million.

- Coca-Cola bought Honest Tea in 2008 for $43 million.

- Nestle bought Tribe Mediterranean Foods in 2008 for $57 million.

- Diamond Foods bought Kettle (Chips) in 2010 for $615 million.

- Post bought Erewhon in 2012, PowerBar in 2014 (from Nestle).

- Campbell Soup Co. bought Wolfgang Puck in 2008, Bolthouse Farms ($1.55 billion) in 2012 and Plum Organics in 2013.

- Hormel Foods bought Applegate Farms in 2015 for $775 million.[15]

With consumer demand for natural, wholesome food and beverage products increasing, food manufacturers have been motivated to replace artificial ingredients, remove chemical additives, eliminate common allergens (MSG, gluten) and use ingredients that have been minimally processed. In response, the food industry has created what they term "clean label" products. The problem for the consumer once again, is that there is no official definition or uniformity as to what "clean label" really means, and that's what makes label reading so cryptic.

I realize that there will always be Pros and Cons regarding specific ingredients and methods of production. If food allergies or sensitivities are involved, then obviously, a deeper and more thorough investigation is called for. For me personally, I've realized I can't know everything about every product, but I can sure do my investigative homework. If per chance, I do come across something that causes an "alert" or piques my interest, I take a deeper look. That way I feel better equipped to make an informed decision about what I want and do not want to include in my diet.

"To eat is a necessity, but to eat intelligently is an art."
– FRANCOIS DE LA ROCHEFOUCAULD

Ultimately, it's up to you how deep and wide you choose to go when it comes to exploring your areas of interest or concern. I've listed a few practices below that have and continue to cause me great concern. They are practices commonly used by the commercial agricultural industry that warrant more attention, education and transparency. These practices include genetic-manipulation, livestock hormone injections and toxic chemicals on farm crops – all occurring without any mandatory monitoring or public disclosure regarding consumer health and safety.

GMOS, GROWTH HORMONES, ANTIBIOTICS AND PESTICIDES

GMOS: Genetic engineering or genetically modifying organisms is the process of taking genes from one species and crossbreeding them into an entirely different species to replicate a desired trait or characteristic. This science falls under the category of modern biotechnology and can sound somewhat innocuous to the uninformed consumer. Not necessarily the case. Some of these so-called "desirable traits" can actually come from a selected virus, bacteria, insect, animal or human gene.

While this technology has proven beneficial in some instances, there has never been – at least for public review – any kind of widespread or rigorous testing concerning the long-term effects of these practices on the human body and the environment.

Let's take the case of a genetically engineered Atlantic salmon. In this case, a growth hormone from a larger Chinook salmon has been introduced to the smaller Atlantic species, resulting in a salmon that grows twice as fast and twice as big. The producing company (Aqua Bounty) says that the fish has the same flavor, texture, color and odor as a regular salmon, but the verdict is out as to whether this fish is *actually* safe for human consumption. As I mentioned, per FDA guidelines, this fish would not have to be labeled as genetically modified. In my estimation, therein lies the problem.

> *There is no requirement in the United States for the agricultural practices and resulting food products containing GMOs, growth hormones, antibiotics, drugs, chemicals, hexane, herbicides and pesticides to be labeled or disclosed to the consumer.*

There have been several animal studies, conducted by the *American Academy of Environmental Medicine* (AAEM), indicating that there are serious health risks associated with genetically modified food. These have included infertility, immune problems, accelerated aging, faulty insulin regulation, impaired organ function and changes in the gastrointestinal system. The AAEM, in their own description, "Is an international association of physicians providing research and education in the recognition, treatment and prevention of illnesses induced by exposures to biological and chemical agents encountered in air, food and water." As a result of the studies conducted by the AAEM, it has been strongly recommended that fellow physicians prescribe healthier, non-GMO foods to their patients.

I've also found the website: the Center for Food Safety (www.CenterForFoodSafety.org) to be a highly informative resource when it comes to recent news, petitions, victories and up to date changes in legislation regarding anything having to do with GMOs.

GROWTH HORMONES: It is thought that at least two-thirds of the beef raised for slaughter in the United States is injected with growth hormones. Growth hormones are injected into an animal to increase its growth, fat and weight for higher market value. The USDA and FDA claim these hormones are safe, but there are legitimate concerns on the part of the consumer that these animal growth hormones could effect their human body in the same way it does animals. This is a reasonable concern, especially when it comes to upsetting the equilibrium of our human body's endocrine system.

Commercial dairy products are mostly procured from cows injected with genetically engineered bovine growth hormone, (rBGH), or recombinant bovine somatotropin (rBST), which unnaturally forces cows to increase their milk production – all in the name of increased revenue.

Despite major opposition from farmers, consumers and scientists, the United States continues to allow dairy farmers to inject their cows with these growth hormones. The FDA approved these Monsanto-developed and manufactured GE hormones in 1993 (essentially a GMO) and they've remained controversial since. As a result, rBGH has since been banned by the European Union, Canada, Australia, Japan, New Zealand and Israel.[16] If a food does not have an *Organic* or *Non-GMO Project Verified* label, then at the least, look for labels stating *No rBGH, rBST* and *No Artificial Hormones*. If you'd like to understand more, a very good and informative website is, the Organic and Non-GMO Report, (www.non-gmoreport.com).

ANTIBIOTICS: 80 percent of all antibiotics sold in the United States goes to chicken, pigs, cows and other animals to stave off the rampant diseases found in the crowded, controlled, factory-farmed animal environment. This is the same animal meat, milk and poultry foods that people generally eat, yet producers are not required to disclose or label the specific drugs, how they're used, on what types of animal and in what quantities – despite growing alarm over human immune dysfunction, allergic reactions and antibiotic resistance. Antibiotic resistance is the ability of a germ or virus to withstand the effects of an antibiotic, thereby reducing or eliminating the effectiveness of that antibiotic."[17]

In its 2013 report, "*Antibiotic Resistance Threats in the United States*," the Centers for Disease Control (CDC) said, "Up to half of antibiotic use in humans and much of antibiotic use in animals is unnecessary and inappropriate and makes everyone less safe."

When shopping, buy certified organic poultry, meat and dairy products, which are free of added growth hormones and antibiotics. Or, buy from small, local farmers whom you can actually ask how they raise and medicate their animals.

PESTICIDES, HERBICIDES AND RODENTICIDES: Doesn't it make sense that the toxic substances applied to food crops and storage warehouses would have a similarly toxic effect on us as well? These substances are meant to kill the bugs, weeds and rodents that cut into food production quotas. The term "-cide" refers to the "act of killing." We would never think of having our fruit and vegetables exposed to rat/rodent poison or ant-and-roach spray – and simply rinse them off before eating, would we? I think not. And yet, these are similar to the toxic substances found within the commercial produce and pre-packaged foods we buy for our family and ourselves.

The same goes for commercially raised animal meats and by-products, for human or pet consumption. Not only is the feed they are ingesting laced with many of these chemicals, but their environments are routinely sprayed as well. Can we assume that if we're eating the meat from these commercially raised animals, we're also taking in these toxic substances? Absolutely. How much is too much? Well, that would depend on how much of your daily diet is from commercially farmed or raised foods versus organic.

As a relatively informed consumer, I've learned to read labels judiciously. I do look for organically labeled foods and non-GMO labeled products. When it comes to certified-organic foods, I feel confident that these foods are produced without pesticides, hormones, antibiotics, irradiation, artificial fertilizers, sewage sludge or genetic modification. Non-GMO, while very important, does *not* have the same stringent, "clean" qualifications that organic does.

	Organic	Non-GMO
No GMO's used:	√	√
No synthetic pesticides used:	√	X
No "Roundup" herbicides used:	√	X
No artificial growth hormones used:	√	X
No excessive antibiotics used:	√	X
No sewage sludge used:	√	X
No Ractopamine drug residue used:	√	X
No neurotoxic Hexane used:	√	X
No food irradiation used:	√	X

Sewage sludge is the mud-like material remaining after treatment of the wastes that flow into local sewage treatment plants. In the U.S., it is estimated that half of treated sewage sludge is applied to farm fields as fertilizer. We're talking sludge that is not purely human waste, but is contaminated with industrial chemicals and household toxic wastes.

Ractopamine is a drug that reduces an animal's fat content and produces more muscle, effectively adding more profit per animal. Ractopamine has been banned in most countries, but for some bewildering reason, the United States, Canada and South Korea consider the meat from Ractopamine-fed livestock as "safe" for human consumption. Unfortunately, along with such harmful additives in one form or another, the animals are also fed genetically engineered feed that is loaded with the potent herbicide glyphosate, which also ends up in the bodies of those eating such meat. Glyphosate is an herbicide that was produced by Monsanto in 1971 and is more commonly known as "Roundup." According to the EPA, it is the most widely used herbicide in the United States with an approximate 100 million pounds per year applied to U.S. farms, parks and lawns. Studies have shown that the glyphosate residues found in genetically engineered foods, such as sugar, corn, soy and wheat – not only cause severe systemic toxicity to those consuming these foods, but they also contribute toward significant nutritional deficiencies.

Hexane has been identified by the FDA as a potent neurotoxin and a carcinogen. It's a chemical by-product of gasoline refining and is also used as a solvent, cleaning agent and in making glue and paint. In the food industry, hexane is used to extract edible oils from seeds and vegetables. Exposure to hexane can affect the central nervous system and cause skin irritations, dizziness, eye redness, nausea, drowsiness, headaches, breathing difficulty, muscle cramps, fatigue and symptoms of peripheral neuropathy in cases of chronic exposure.

I've found it to be practical and wise on my part to familiarize myself with the commercially processed foods that contain one or more of the most commonly bio-engineered food crops. Unless a food or product in one of the following categories is labeled as certified-organic or non-GMO, then you can assume it's been genetically-engineered – and best avoided.

Here are some of the statistics:

- 94 percent of all soy is genetically engineered.

- 90 percent of all canola is genetically engineered.

- 88 percent of all corn is genetically engineered. (Excluding blue corn).

- 90 percent of all cotton is genetically engineered. (Cottonseed oil).

- 95 percent of all sugar beets are genetically engineered (Used for white sugar).

- 50 percent or more of all Hawaiian papaya is genetically-engineered.[18]

Part Six
Therapeutic Supplements

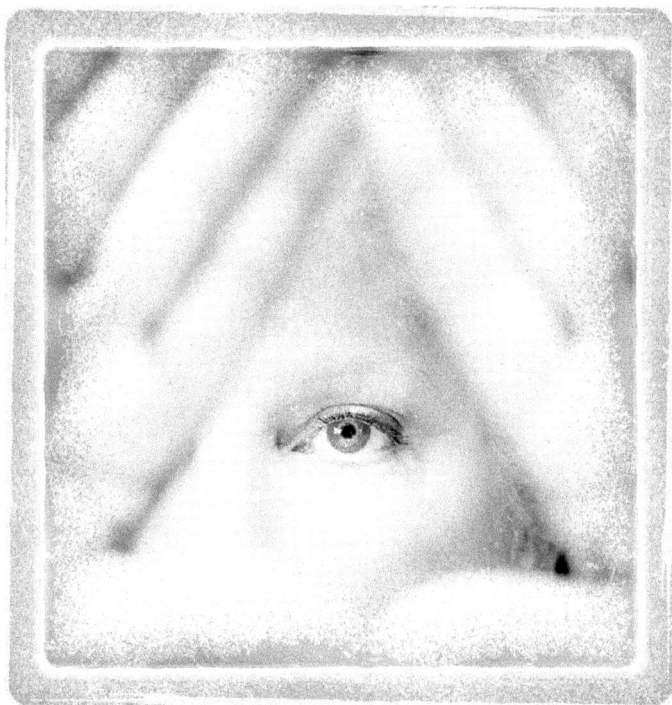

"*A path is made by walking on it.*"
~ CHUANG TZU

21

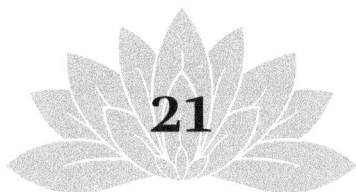

Cherry-Picking Supplements

How do you know which supplements are best? The simple answer is: the ones you feel a difference with. What's effective for one person is not necessarily suited for the next. Nutritional and biochemical individuality is influenced and determined by a person's unique genetics, lifestyle, diet, health, age and environment. These days, we're exposed to every kind of health product, dietary program and social media marketing blitz imaginable – all touting ways to have a healthier body, a clearer mind and a more youthful appearance.

The way I tend to look at supplements is as added insurance – an enhancement to my already healthy diet and lifestyle. While many of us strive to eat a predominantly balanced, organic, whole foods diet most of the time, there are going to be those unforeseen times when our lives have us running at a deficit. That's when it helps to have some extra "supplemental" insurance.

When it comes to the "cleanest" and most effective supplements, I've found it best to go with the food-based, bio-available ones that contain therapeutic dosages.

A good place to start is with a well-rounded (food-based) multi-vitamin/mineral/enzyme supplement. You can then add whatever additional supplements you desire, alongside the multi. Besides my chosen multi, I typically add a super-food grass, greens and algae powder, magnesium and iodine minerals, omega-3, vitamin D3 and probiotics – all depending upon my circumstances and how I'm feeling. Sometimes it's hard to know if supplements are really working, especially if you feel OK most of the time. The only way I've been able to get a true read is to *not* take them for a day and see if I notice a difference. The times I've chosen to do that, I have definitely noticed a difference – like there's a big energetic hole in the bucket – and I'm running at a deficit. I've also discovered a few chosen immunity-building combos for when my resistance feels compromised. They will typically nip anything in the proverbial bud.

Listed below are some of the supplements I have found to be effective in keeping the body healthy and resilient. You'll find as your health, lifestyle, circumstances and environment change, so will your diet, supplementation and activity.

When contemplating the specific type, strength or form of supplementation best suited for you, it's always beneficial to do your homework regarding product effectiveness, company reputation and any possible contraindications. If you have any questions or concerns, chat with a knowledgeable nutritional consultant or your preferred Eastern or Western medical professional.

Chlorella and Spirulina, Barley Grass, Wheat Grass and Oat Grass: These green super-food algae and organic grasses provide an astounding amount of nutrients. They nourish us on a cellular level, supporting all bodily systems: muscular,

skeletal, skin, nervous, respiratory, hormonal, cardiovascular, circulatory, digestive, reproductive and immune
systems. They assist the various bodily systems to run at
peak efficiency with optimal energy production, especially
when combined with other nutritive factors. When ingested,
these chlorophyll-rich cereal grasses and micro-algae have
a remarkable resemblance to our own blood composition,
acting as an essential life-blood and life force infusion. They
help cleanse, oxygenate and detoxify the blood.

> *Chlorophyll is considered plant "blood." It is almost*
> *identical in composition to our own blood cells.*
> *Chlorophyll produces the green pigment in all plants. It*
> *is known to strengthen immunity, reduce inflammation,*
> *and cleanse, alkalize and oxygenate our blood.*

They also help promote healthy flora throughout the digestive system – boosting our immunity and alkalizing our
pH. When mixed into any juice, smoothie or shake, these
super-food powders can have a tremendous impact on
our energy level and overall vitality. My personal favorite
nutrient-dense food product is *Green Vibrance*. It's a potent
assortment of organic cereal grasses, algae, whole-food
veggie concentrates, seaweeds, medicinal herbs, probiotics,
anti-aging antioxidants, micronutrients and enzymes. I've
been using this super-food powder since the mid '90s and
have found over the years that the company has continually
reformulated and improved its original formula. It is pres-
ently on version 14.1. (Green Vibrance by Vibrant Health.)

Transfer Factor: A balanced immune system is vital to our
health and well-being. I have found this supplement to be
highly effective whenever my immunity feels compromised

or I've been exposed to someone who is not feeling well. I will typically keep a bottle in my purse for those unexpected encounters – and to offer those around me who might be "coming down with something." I find it especially effective when taken at bedtime, while the body has some time to rest and recuperate. I think of transfer factors as an extremely effective and natural antibiotic, antibacterial and antimicrobial – and have found it especially useful for those who are routinely antibiotic resistant.

Transfer factors are described as tiny messenger molecules that actually transfer "immune memory and knowledge" from the more healthy functioning immune cells to the weakened, more vulnerable ones. They provide intelligence from one bodily system to another, by first identifying any invading microorganisms (germs), and then building and strengthening immunity to prevent the germs from taking hold. They literally aid the immune system in best recognizing, responding to and remembering potential threats and stressors.

Typically transfer factors are sourced from the "ultra-filtration" of bovine colostrum and egg yolks. The cellular, immune memory and knowledge is provided by the mother's immune system to her baby – for recognizing and warding off outside threats. Transfer factors were first discovered in 1949 by the American immunologist Dr. H. Sherwood Lawrence, (1916 – 2004). (4-Life Transfer Factor).

Yin Chiao: (pronounced Yin Chow) is a traditional Chinese herbal remedy used to combat the symptoms of the common head cold and imbalances that come with the change of season. It is especially effective at the onset of a cold, say the first 12-24 hours, when Yin, watery symptoms are just beginning. I have found it to be highly assistive in helping to shorten the time period of symptoms, as well as helping to strengthen and nourish the body's immune system. I've also taken it as a preventative, prior to meeting with someone who has recently had a head cold. It does seem to minimize any exposure.

Wellness Formula: I have used this formula on and off for many years. I find it to be most useful at the first sign of a cough, cold, sore throat or chest tightness, as well as when symptoms of "susceptibility" first occur and the body's natural defenses are down. It's a powerful combination of vitamins, antioxidants and traditional, immune-enhancing herbs, such as astragalus, isatis, echinacea and garlic, that helps the body cleanse, detox and fortify. When caught early enough, one day of continual dosing will usually do the trick. This formula is not typically taken as a daily supplement, but rather as a supportive tonic when feeling stressed or when immunity becomes compromised. (Wellness Formula. Source Naturals).

Omega-3 Essential Fatty Acids: After introducing Omega-3 acids into my diet, I noticed a marked increase in the moisture and pliability of my skin. I also felt a clarity and sharpness within my mind. It was really quite remarkable, as compared to how I felt before taking them. I thought I was getting enough Omega-3s from other vegetarian sources (flax, walnuts, chia), but the addition of marine algae proved unparalleled. I've come to understand that our brain uses a complex nerve network to send messages and communicate with every bodily system for optimal function and effectiveness.

Omega-3 fatty acids actually cover or coat those nerve endings, allowing for better synapse messaging, as well as supporting the body's regenerative capabilities and energy. They've also been shown to assist and ease the symptoms of depression and anxiety. Omega-3s are typically sourced from fish oil, krill, marine algae, flaxseeds and nuts. I personally use a vegan source derived from marine algae. (Nuique. Omega-3).

Magnesium: It's estimated that up to 80 percent of Americans are deficient in the essential mineral magnesium. This is not only due to the nutrient depleted soil in which our food grows, but also because of processed/sugary foods, carbonated sodas, municipally-treated water, prescription medications and poor nutrient absorption within the gut. I started taking magnesium to help with foot cramping during yoga postures. It made quite a difference. It also helps tremendously with fatigued muscles after a day of intense hiking, unaccustomed physical labor, yard-work or gardening. Magnesium has been shown to have a relaxing effect on smooth muscles and has proven effective in any condition involving the tightening and cramping of muscles. These would include all muscle-contracting conditions such as headaches, hypertension, dysmenorrhea, constipation, asthma and heart complications.

It was an epiphany many years ago when I first realized that the Epsom salt baths I'd always taken to relax my muscles were actually magnesium salts (magnesium sulfate).

Virtually all bodily systems rely on magnesium for at least some of their metabolic functions. It's been shown to boost white blood cell production, enhance enzymatic function, reduce inflammation and detoxify the body.

Magnesium is one of the most powerful anti-inflammatories out there. Not only is it used in helping to relax muscles, it is critically important for a deep and restful sleep.

There are many forms of magnesium on the market today. The most bioavailable and absorbable oral form tends to be magnesium glycinate. Other forms that have been proven bioavailable and effective are magnesium carbonate, citrate, taurate and malate. Magnesium oil is also quite effective when applied topically. Not really an oil per se, "magnesium oil" is actually a highly concentrated solution of magnesium chloride in water. It is applied to the skin, as any topical oil would be.

Organic, chlorophyll-rich, green leafy vegetables such as spinach and Swiss chard are excellent sources of magnesium, as are pumpkin seeds, flax seeds, almonds, tempeh, sesame seeds, quinoa, sunflower seeds, cocoa powder, chlorella and spirulina. Coconut water is also high in magnesium.

Vitamin D3: Vitamin D has long been considered an essential nutrient for keeping organs healthy and fully functional. Vitamin D is not actually what we think of as a "regular" vitamin, but rather a steroidal hormone precursor that we get from sun exposure or supplementation. It wasn't until I investigated deeper the attributes of Vitamin D, (in particular vitamin D3) and its effect on our health and well-being that I understood its critical importance. People with optimum Vitamin D levels can expect better health across the board.

This nutrient has been shown to boost the immune system function, improve cardiovascular health, protect against autoimmunity and play a role in both mood and metabolic rate, resulting in a longer and healthier life, fewer diseases, stronger bones and muscles, fewer infections, fewer headaches, and less depression, pain and inflammation.

The most natural way to obtain Vitamin D is from the sun. This is why you see people getting what is called seasonal depression (SAD – seasonal affect disorder) during the winter months when sun exposure is at a minimum. As our exposure to the sun is reduced, our Vitamin D levels are equally reduced. It's a good idea to take a combo supplement of Vitamin D with Vitamin K2, as it helps the body to utilize calcium more efficiently while mineralizing bones and joints. A number of companies combine the two supplements into one capsule.

> *Vitamin D has been known to boost immune function, reduce inflammation, optimize bodyweight and help reverse depression.*

I personally take a minimum of 5,000 mg per day of Vitamin D3, and have for many years. My 91 year old mother has also taken 5,000 mg. per day for many years with great success. In each of our blood panels, there are no contraindications and our Vitamin D levels repeatedly register in the "normal" range.

Whole Food-Based, Multi-Supplement: When you are eating well, a multiple's first and foremost purpose is as back-up insurance to supply the nutrients that may be running low or lacking. A good, effective whole-food "multi" includes vitamins, minerals, antioxidants, tonic herbs and the particularly important phyto-nutrients from super food algae such as spirulina, chlorella and cereal grass sprouts or extracts. These are more readily absorbed and utilized by the body than most of our table foods. These comprehensive nutrients help to promote cellular health and regeneration and provide stabilized energy reserves for handling life's ever-changing daily stressors. (Life Essence™ by Pure Essence Lab).

Ashwagandha (Winter Cherry): Ashwagandha is a popular adaptogenic herb used in Ayurvedic medicine, proven to be highly effective in relieving anxiety, tension and stress-induced, adrenal fatigue. It has been shown to lower cortisol levels and assist in balancing thyroid hormones. Cortisol is activated by caffeine, stress and sugar. When cortisol levels are continually triggered by any of these factors, we end up with our sympathetic nervous system in overdrive. This depleting cycle not only causes adrenal fatigue, but compromised immunity, premature aging and exhausted energy supplies.

One of the greatest things about adaptogens is that they adjust and adapt to our bodily needs. With Ashwagandha, its adaptogenic properties help to naturally balance our hormones, whether they are overactive, sluggish or fatigued.

Ashwagandha is considered the Ayurvedic equivalent to ginseng and can prove overly stimulating, especially when taken at or near bedtime. (Ashwagandha Root by Organic India).

Ashwagandha is one of the most powerful herbs in Ayurvedic healing. It is traditionally known for its restorative properties, for strengthening the immune system and for helping to relieve anxiety, tension and stress-induced, adrenal fatigue.

Iodine: Iodine is a naturally occurring mineral found in seawater and soil. It is best known for its role in suitable thyroid-hormone production, but is also essential for healthfully balancing all hormones within the body. Hormones basically "run the show" when it comes to our bodily functions.

Iodine is found within every cell of the body and is especially concentrated in the glandular or endocrine system. It is utilized by every hormone receptor and when deficient, can often be a contributing factor in hormonal imbalance and dysfunction. Iodine deficiencies have been known to contribute to conditions such as fibrocystic breast and ovarian disease, thyroid imbalances, autoimmune diseases, prostate disorders and abnormal blood sugar levels in the body.[19]

> *Nascent (atomic) iodine is recognized by the body as the same form that the thyroid produces for the creation of T3 and T4 – and is found to be easily absorbed and utilized.*

Iodine can be found naturally in seaweeds and seafood and also through supplementation. I've personally used two kinds of oral supplementation: a pill that contains iodide and iodine (Iodoral™) and a tincture made from nascent or atomic iodine (Magnascent™).

Nascent iodine is an electrically charged form of iodine, and is the very same form as the thyroid produces for the creation of T3 and T4 hormones. I personally feel a difference with the nascent iodine, as compared with the Iodoral. There's a tangible feeling of "aliveness" in my body and mind with the nascent iodine that I don't experience with the Iodoral. As I've said, supplementation is an individual thing, and you've just got to experiment with different ones to see what works best for you. I also do a fair amount of seaweed, especially dulse tabs (Bernard Jensen) that give me an extra iron and mineral boost.

> "All of the glands of the body depend on adequate iodine levels to function optimally."
> - DAVID BROWNSTEIN MD

The typical dose of Iodoral™ (by Optimox) tends to be one 12.5mg tablet to maintain healthy iodine levels. This is close to the same level found in the seafood and seaweed-rich diets of the Okinawan people, written about in Chapter 7.

The nascent or atomic iodine is reputed to be the most bioavailable and the least toxic and irritating of all the iodine formulas available. Studies have indicated that the electrically charged nascent form of iodine is able to easily enter and saturate the thyroid without any toxic buildup. Plus, it is readily recognized and absorbed into the body, much like the T3 and T4 hormones naturally produced by the thyroid.[20]

Probiotics: Probiotics are the beneficial bacterial strains in the intestinal tract that promote effective digestion, nutrient absorption and support a healthy immune system. Our healthy intestinal micro-flora is affected by stress, caffeine, alcohol, sugary/processed foods and prescription medications. Daily probiotic intake can help support immune function, alleviate gastrointestinal strain, relieve skin conditions and reduce harmful bacteria, yeast infections and allergies. They are especially helpful when used in conjunction with prescription antibiotics. You can incorporate probiotics into your diet in either supplement or food form. Fermented foods, such as sauerkraut, miso, pickles, tempeh, kim-chi, kombucha tea and plain unflavored yogurt and kefir, are all good, natural sources of probiotics.

Probiotics improve immunity, nutrient absorption, digestion, inflammation, elimination, detoxification and antibiotic efficacy. Eighty percent of our immune system is located in the digestive system.

Digestive Aids and Enzymes: Digestive enzymes function as biological catalysts in breaking down food, improving both our digestive function and nutrient absorption. The primary digestive enzymes are protease (to digest protein), amylase (to digest carbohydrates), cellulase (to breakdown fiber), lactase (to digest milk sugar), lipase (to digest fat) and maltase (to convert grain's complex sugars into useable blood sugar). The body naturally produces sufficient enzymes to maintain optimum levels of health. However, as our bodies age, along with experiencing life's daily stressors, the body's production of enzymes decrease, which effects digestion and absorption of nutrients.

Increasing the amount of raw, organic, unprocessed foods you eat will assist in supplying your body with the enzymes it needs. Eating in a relaxed manner, chewing your food well and eating smaller, more frequent meals, contributes greatly in supporting a healthy digestive system.

Apple Cider Vinegar: Apple cider vinegar dates back as far as 400 B.C. when Hippocrates purportedly used this multi-purpose remedy to effectively treat his patients. It's so much more than *simply* a condiment. I have used this for years and found it to be one of the most effective health tonics around. It is known to have antibacterial, antiseptic, anti-inflammatory and anti-fungal properties, making it highly beneficial for a multitude of ailments. These would include intestinal bloating and gas, skin irritations, sore throat gargle, as well as inflammation of joints. It has become my preferred facial astringent because its pH is so perfectly suited for the skin. I've used it as an after-wash hair rinse, as it removes remaining product residue, leaving my hair shiny and clean. I've also found it to be highly effective as a body, joint, muscle and skin detox, when added directly into a bath (half to whole quart bottle). It is absolutely one of my favorite "go to" products.

Make sure to get the organic, unfiltered and raw version of apple cider vinegar, that contains the "mother" culture, filled with friendly bacteria and enzymes. (Braggs).

I have discovered a great summer balancing-tonic, using the following ingredients:

- 1 glass filtered water 10-12 oz.
- 1+ Tbsps. organic apple cider vinegar
- 1+ Tbsps. organic lemon juice
- 1 tsp. to 1 Tbsp. maple syrup or coconut sugar, if sweetening is desired.
- I also will add about a ½ teaspoon of organic cinnamon or organic ginger powder, on occasion, depending on mood and utility. Use a whisk to blend.

"If you get the inside right, the outside will
fall into place."
- ECKHART TOLLE

" *Just trust yourself*
and then you will know
how to live."

~ GOETHE

EPILOGUE

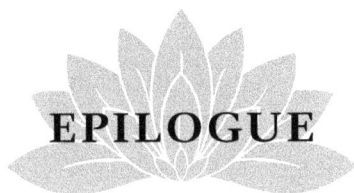

Living the Life

Whenever we embark upon a journey of self-discovery, we are given an opportunity to observe, evaluate and often times reconsider our very-comfortable, habituated patterns of thinking, eating, living and behaving.

It's in activating our inner intelligence that we create a renewed and revitalized way of thinking and living – one that allows us to experience vibrant health, balanced living, dynamic energy, enhanced moods and a satisfying, enjoyable life.

> "You have all the tools you need to access your pure potential, to evolve your dreams into reality, and to live a life of extraordinary design."
> – DEEPAK CHOPRA

This particular path of self-discovery gives you the practical wisdom and awareness to become harmoniously balanced, in your body, mind and emotions by adjusting your diet, lifestyle, attitude and environment.

With a simple bit of practice you'll begin to experience a more heightened awareness of your body and temperament. By implementing the specific practices, activities and dietary choices best suited for your unique nature – you are proactively contributing towards your "Highest and Best Self." It is the best investment you will ever make.

Does this shift in awareness happen overnight? Usually not. But it's been said by many a behavioral scientist, that it takes about 21 days to create a new habit and eliminate the old. I can attest to this. My experience confirms that if you invest yourself earnestly in this practice for 21 consecutive days, you will absolutely reprogram your mind and body. Truth.

It's really what this whole journey is about – reconnecting with your internal wisdom.

It's there for the asking...

> "You are what your deep, driving desire is.
> As your desire is, so is your will.
> As your will is, so is your deed.
> As your deed is, so is your destiny."
> - THE BRIHADARANYAKA UPANISHAD

This is a path of incremental awakening that takes time, intention, awareness and practice. There's a direct connection between how much intention, passion and focus we direct toward something – *anything* – and how fast it comes to fruition. It's one of the most satisfying feelings in the world to experience the power and command of creating your life the way you want. There's really nothing quite like it.

As we progress down our individually unique, evolutionary path, it's clear to see that being healthy and well adjusted is so much more than just a dietary approach, belief system or protocol. It's an ever-changing blend of desire, curiosity, instincts, passion, exploration and full-on engagement with lighting up the circuitry within our wonderfully accessible, "instinctive self."

Once that happens, our body, mind, spirit and life become an enlivening, tuned-in and turned-on experience. I have personally found it to be the most engaging, empowering and fulfilling path there is.

> "The Journey is the Reward."
> – TAOIST PROVERB

With great appreciation to you, dear reader, I thank you for traveling this way with me. You are my greatest inspiration in creating and delivering this book.

May you always feel supported, encouraged and inspired on your own journey toward health, happiness and awakening.

My Heart to Yours...
This is The Beginning of
Anything You Desire...

NOTES

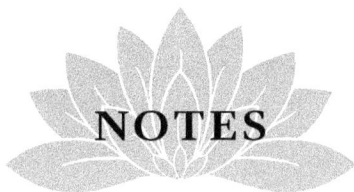

1. Physis Comes In From The Cold Author: Dr Rashid Bhikha. Published: *Journal of Natural Medicine* – Issue 20 Oct/Nov 2005.

2. Ronald E. Kotzsch, PhD (Harvard, 1981) "Macrobiotics Yesterday and Today". (Japan Publications, NY, 1985) Chapter 2: Sagen Ishizuka: the Founder of Modern Macrobiotics."

3. *Mind-Body-Green Newsletter,* By Emi Boscamp 1/5/2015 "It was by implementing Ishizuka's, ...yin-yang concepts of a balanced, whole-foods diet, exercise, simple living, and being in touch with nature, society, and oneself...that Ohsawa's health was reclaimed."

4. What is Fortified Flour? Healthy Eating. SF Gate. by Sukhsatej Batra, Demand Media.

5. Farm Use of Antibiotics Defies Scrutiny. *New York Times.* Sept. 3, 2012. By Sabrina Tavernise.

6. *Journal of Applied Nutrition* 1993; 45:35-39. Organic foods vs. supermarket foods: Element Levels Synopsis: Over a 2 year period, organically and conventionally grown apples, potatoes, pears, wheat and sweet corn were purchased in the western suburbs of Chicago and analyzed for mineral content. Four to 15 samples were taken for each food group. On a per-weight basis, average levels of essential minerals were much higher in the organically grown food than in the conventionally grown food. The organically grown food averaged 63% higher in calcium,

78% higher in chromium, 73% higher in iron, 118% higher in magnesium, 178% higher in molybdenum, 91% higher in phosphorus, 125% higher in potassium and 60% higher in zinc. The organically raised food averaged 29% lower in mercury than the conventionally raised food.

7. Caloric restriction. In 1934, Mary Crowell and Clive McCay of Cornell University conducted a landmark nutritional study with rats. They discovered that rats fed a diet with 30% reduced calories (while maintaining their vital nutrient levels) lived up to twice as long as their counterparts that ate as much as they wanted. (pg. 67, bottom) More recently, former UCLA professor and pathologist Roy Walford, MD and his student, Richard Weindruch, conducted a similar experiment with mice. They found that the group with a drastically reduced caloric intake doubled their lifespan, when compared to mice that ate a normal diet. These calorie-restricted mice also had higher energy levels and a significant delay in all age-related diseases. Not long after that, *Life Extension* magazine published an article by Donald K. Ingram, Mark A. Lane and George S. Roth about caloric restriction in our nearest genetic relatives, the primates. The study found that when monkeys consumed 30% fewer calories, they lived 30% longer, reaching 32 years of age, which corresponds to 96 human years. That's the equivalent of adding 21 years to the normal human life expectancy of 75. "The 9 Steps to Keep the Doctor Away: Simple Actions to Shift Your Body and Mind to Optimum Health and Greater Longevity." By Dr. Rashid Buttar. June 1, 2010

8. *60 Minutes,* "Mt. Athos, A Visit to the Holy Mountain," aired on April 24, 2011. "A Foolproof Anti-Cancer Diet, with Just One or Two Drawbacks," Sunday London Times, December 7, 2007.

9. *The Yellow Emperor's Classic of Medicine* (the Neijing Suwen) ~240 B.C. translated by Maoshing Ni, Shambala Publications ISBN 1-57062-080-6 © 1995 further edited by Paul Farago.

10. Dr. William Davis, The author of *Wheat Belly* wrote, "Modern wheat has been hybridized (crossing different strains to generate new characteristics; 5% of proteins generated in the offspring, for instance, are not present in either parent), backcrossed (repeated crossing to winnow out a specific

trait, e.g., short stature), and hybridized with non-wheat plants (to introduce entirely unique genes). In common usage, of course, hybridization simply means mating two plants or animals to generate a unique offspring. I am no defender of genetic-modification, but it is pure craziness that Agribusiness apologists defend modern wheat because it is not yet the recipient of "genetic modification." ("wheatbellyblog. com/2012/02/Wheat-is-not-genetically-modified.)

11. *Why the Rise in Gluten Sensitivity?* (CBS News). Modern wheat is a "perfect, chronic poison," according to Dr. William Davis, a cardiologist who has published a book all about the world's most popular grain. Davis said that the wheat we eat these days isn't the wheat your grandma had: "It's an 18-inch tall plant created by genetic research in the '60s and '70s," he said on "CBS This Morning." "This thing has many new features nobody told you about, such as there's a new protein in this thing called gliadin. It's not gluten. I'm not addressing people with gluten sensitivities and celiac disease. I'm talking about everybody else because everybody else is susceptible to the gliadin protein that is an opiate. This thing binds into the opiate receptors in your brain and in most people stimulates appetite, such that we consume 440 more calories per day, 365 days per year." Asked if the farming industry could change back to the grain it formerly produced, Davis said it could, but it would not be economically feasible because it yields less per acre. However, Davis said a movement has begun with people turning away from wheat and dropping substantial weight. "If three people lost eight pounds, big deal," he said. "But we're seeing hundreds of thousands of people losing 30, 80, 150 pounds."

12. *The Journal of Clinical Endocrinology and Metabolism.* 2009 May; Epub 2009 Feb 17.

13. Caffeine Database. CaffeineInformer.com. Overcaffeinated.org.

14. *Natural Society News.* 'Foods with Hidden Animal Products.' By Elizabeth Renter. 8/29/14. Desiblitz. 'Animal Ingredients in Vegetarian Foods.' By Nazhat Khan. 6/27/10.

  * Red Juices, candies, applesauce and popsicles: A red colorant known as carmine, cochineal, carminic acid, Crimson Lake,

Natural Red 4, C.I. 75470, or E120, actually comes from a ground-up beetle. Dannon uses (or has used) crushed beetles (carmine) in their yogurts.

* Marshmallows, Jell-O, gummy-bears, Starbursts, Altoids, Jelly Beans, Pastilles, Trident sugar-free gum and some brands of sour cream and non-fat yogurt all contain gelatin. Gelatin is a protein derived from animal bones, tendons, cartilage and skin.

* Beer – Many beer-makers, including Guinness, use something called Isinglass, which is a gelatin from fish bladders. (Beer makers also use gelatin in their brews).

* Berry-flavored foods – Castoreum is considered a "natural flavor," so many food makers don't go beyond labeling it as such in the ingredient's list. However, this flavor is derived from the anal glands of beavers. Yep, this really happens.

* Food products with Omega – Be cautious of any foods that advertise added Omega-3 fats. The source is often times fish oil. In the case of Smart Balance, Otria Greek Yogurt Dip or Tropicana's Heart Health with Omega-3 orange juice, the added Omega's are all from fish oil.

* Worcestershire sauce – Worcestershire is made with anchovies. Commonly used to season meat, Worcestershire sauce is often added to veggie-dishes, tofu and tempeh as a savory sauce by well-intended, but unknowing cooks. If a savory sauce is served, ask whether it contains Worcestershire sauce. Cesar salad dressing, olive tapenade and pasta puttanesca sauce often times contain anchovies.

* Cheese – Many cheeses contain rennet, made from the stomach lining of calves. Vegetable rennet or microbial enzymes are the commonly preferred vegetarian substitute.

* Foods and food additives with animal content. Many foods have hidden animal ingredients. Barbecue Baked Lays potato chips include chicken in their 'natural flavors'. Tortillas, refried beans, baked beans, split pea soup, cornbread mix, piecrusts, French fries and cupcakes can typically contain lard or animal fat as an ingredient.

15. *Business Insider.* 8/27/2014 Drake Baer. "19" Local And National Natural Brands Owned by Giant Corporations. Cornucopia Institute, Dr. Phil Howard 2/13 "Who Owns Organic."

16. *Food Safety – From the Farm to the Fork.* Report on Public Health Aspects of the Use of Bovine Somatotrophin - 15-16 March 1999

17. *Farm Use of Antibiotics Defies Scrutiny.* Sabrina Tavernise Sept. 3, 2012.

18. Institute for Responsible Technology. Copyright © 2006-2014. Jeffrey M. Smith.

19. Role of lipid peroxidation and oxidative stress in the association between thyroid diseases and breast cancer. *Critical Reviews in Oncology/Hematology,* Volume 68, Issue 2, Pages 107-114 M. Gago-Dominguez, J. Castelao.

20. Nascent Iodine, "Iodine, Why You Need It and Why You Can't Live Without It." David Brownstein, MD.

www.ingramcontent.com/pod-product-compliance
Lightning Source LLC
Chambersburg PA
CBHW062207270326
41930CB00009B/1674